The Mindful
Mom-to-Be

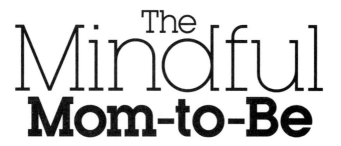

The Mindful Mom-to-Be

A MODERN DOULA'S GUIDE TO BUILDING A HEALTHY FOUNDATION FROM PREGNANCY THROUGH BIRTH

LORI BREGMAN

with Stefani Newman

FOREWORD BY MOLLY SIMS

RODALE.

© 2015 by Lori Bregman

All rights reserved. No part of this publication may be reproduced or transmitted in any form or by any means, electronic or mechanical, including photocopying, recording, or any other information storage and retrieval system, without the written permission of the publisher.

Rodale books may be purchased for business or promotional use or for special sales. For information, please write to:
Special Markets Department, Rodale, Inc., 733 Third Avenue, New York, NY 10017

Printed in the United States of America

Rodale Inc. makes every effort to use acid-free ♾, recycled paper ♻.

Illustrations by David M. Gutiérrez

Book design by Christina Gaugler

Library of Congress Cataloging-in-Publication Data is on file with the publisher

ISBN 978–1–62336–301–7 paperback

Distributed to the trade by Macmillan

4 6 8 10 9 7 5 3   paperback

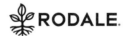

We inspire and enable people to improve their lives and the world around them.

rodalebooks.com

For all mindful moms and moms-to-be

CONTENTS

FOREWORD

I worked with Lori during my entire pregnancy with my son Brooks. It was a difficult pregnancy with a fear that went so deep because I just wanted my baby to be okay. She was with me every step of the way. Every step I took, I felt safe knowing that what I was doing was helping my baby.

Lori was my complete body, mind, and spirit support system from prepregnancy into new mommyhood. Her bodywork, transformative yoga, breathwork, and meditations helped calm me, ground me, and connect me with my baby when he was in the womb, while the monthly recipes she provided helped me focus not only on how to feed myself, but also on how to nourish my baby at each stage of development.

Lori's program provided me with the tools, insight, and wisdom to journey into a new life phase, learning how to be more present and mindful. Lori made the 9 months a beautiful experience. She was truly my Bible throughout my pregnancy, birth, and beyond. I am now blessed with baby number 2 on the way, and once again Lori is by my side, supporting me every step of the way. *The Mindful Mom-to-Be* will give you the knowledge, peace of mind, and clarity you need to have a happy and healthy pregnancy, as well as the tools you need to transition into motherhood.

—Molly Sims

INTRODUCTION

Congratulations! I am so excited for you. Pregnancy may be one of the most magical, exciting, confusing, stressful, and transformative times in a woman's life. Over the next few months, your little one will be growing and developing inside of you. He or she will be as much a part of you as your lungs, heart, or kidneys. Just as a caterpillar becomes a butterfly, you are morphing into something new as well—you'll not only give birth to a baby, you'll also birth a part of yourself that never existed before—a mother. You're already starting to parent your child as you take care of yourself during pregnancy, and the healthier, happier, and calmer you are, the healthier, happier, and calmer your baby will be.

I'm a pregnancy coach and birth doula, offering complete mind and body support before and during pregnancy, birth, and the first year after birth. My pregnancy-coaching program, Rooted for Life, helps build a solid and healthy foundation for moms and babies to grow from. I also offer an in-depth doula program for clients. I've worked with hundreds of women and helped countless children come into this world, and I've never seen two women or babies experience pregnancy, labor, and birth the same way. It's my belief that there is no right or only way to do this—but there is a right way for you, your child, and your family. You just need to find, create, trust, and follow that way—and I'm here to help you.

These days, doulas are a very popular choice among women to help with pregnancy and childbirth, as well as the postpartum period. Doulas are not a new concept; we've been working with pregnant women since ancient times! Finally, mainstream medicine is catching up with the idea and importance of having someone else, aside from a doctor or nurse, by a woman's side to help support her mind, body, *and* spirit throughout pregnancy and beyond. The word *doula* comes from an ancient Greek word meaning "woman servant" or "caregiver." (I prefer the latter!) Doulas can help you birth your baby at home, at a birthing center, or in a hospital, with or without pain medication—even if you have a C-section, a doula can help wherever or however you choose to have your baby.

WHAT DO DOULAS DO?

Birth doulas can:

- Prepare and educate both you and your partner for pregnancy and birth

- Create a unique birth plan that supports your wishes for labor and delivery

- Stay by your side during labor and delivery, supporting you throughout the entire birth process

- Coach and guide you through any emotional blocks or fears that might come up during birth

- Create a safe and peaceful space with their energy, candles, aromatherapy, and music

- Use massage, visualizations, meditation, breathwork, energy work, sounding, and movement to help with pain management and comfort

- Advocate for the mother and her partner and help facilitate better communication between the mother and her caregiver

- Reduce the possibility of Caesarean section

Ever since I can remember, I've been drawn to working with pregnant women, new mothers, and children. Over the past 28 years, I've studied all types of holistic healing, from yoga, energy work, intuition, bodywork, chakras, herbal healing, aromatherapy, meditation, spiritual guidance, breathwork, and the mind/body connection to the healing properties of food and more. As a healer, I've traveled all over the world to work with celebrities, producers, directors, talent agents, rock stars, writers, billionaires, and CEOs, but my greatest joy and passion is working with pregnant women. There is nothing more rewarding than helping to bring a child into this world.

- Reduce the need for pain medication and epidurals
- Minimize the length of labor
- Calm anxiety and reduce depression
- Help with confidence and self-esteem

Postpartum doulas can:

- Provide breastfeeding and bonding support
- Help with house chores, light cleaning, errands, and cooking
- Share information about baby care and infant massage
- Nurture, massage, and care for the mother
- Help care for the baby so you can rest, eat, and shower

What doulas *don't* do:

- Doulas are *not* medical professionals. They don't perform medical exams or tasks, diagnose conditions, or deliver babies.
- Doulas do not project their views onto you, and they should *never* judge you or make you feel bad about the choices and decisions you make.

It's my belief that before we are born, we choose our parents and have a soul contract with them. My own birth was something I had to work back through spiritually and emotionally in order to understand my authentic self. My mother was young and unmarried when she had me. She was in denial about her pregnancy, went into a major depression, and considered putting me up for adoption. Her labor and delivery were traumatic experiences. She labored alone, as my dad and family members weren't allowed in the room, was put to sleep before I was pulled from her, and was then prevented from seeing or holding me for days afterward, as I lay in an incubator. My mom cried as she explained all of this to me, and said, "Lori, the fact that you survived that pregnancy—your soul was meant to be here."

Things were very different back then, and we still have a long way to go in how we help women approach and handle labor and birth. I love my parents beyond words. They did the best they could given what they knew at the time, especially being so young. My greatest wound turned out to be my greatest gift: Out of my own healing, life path, studying, and deep passion, my pregnancy-coaching and doula practice, Rooted for Life, was born! I share the tools and wisdom from my journey with others so they, too, can be transformed into whole and empowered people. I combine spiritual and intuitive life coaching and healing work with the practicalities of dealing with pregnancy. I believe that the more supported women are, the better they will feel during their pregnancies and the happier, healthier, and more at peace they will be as mothers—and the happier their babies will be, too!

You can use this book any way you like. Every chapter touches on a mindful theme for you to work on for that month, something important I believe all women can explore to help birth themselves into mindful, healthy, and happy moms. The chapters proceed chronologically through pregnancy, labor, and delivery. I'll walk you through what's happening with your body during each month and give you a peek into how your baby is growing and changing. I also offer many natural remedies, tips, and tricks for dealing with pregnancy ailments and concerns. We can't change what we aren't aware of, so I've planted lots of little seeds throughout this book to help raise your awareness and consciousness and to bring you closer to feeling like a mindful mom.

Some things I say throughout this book might resonate with you, and some might not. Pick out what *you feel* is right for you, and work with it. If a certain theme doesn't interest you and another one does, practice that for the month. You can always go back to the first idea at another time, even after you deliver your baby. Strengthening your own foundation is one of the very best beginnings you can give your child. We lead by example: Children watch, mimic, absorb, and become what *we* are. The healthier, happier, and more consciously and mindfully we live our lives, the more our children will as well. It all starts with you.

CHAPTER 1

Month One

HEALTHY MOM, HEALTHY BABY

"A house must be built on solid foundations if it is to last. The same principle applies to man, otherwise he too will sink back into the soft ground and become swallowed up by the world of illusion."

—**Sai Baba**

If you ask any mom-to-be her greatest wish for her children, the first thing she'll say is, "I want them to be healthy!" Of course, some circumstances surrounding the health of our children are beyond our control. But there are many things you can absolutely do to make sure your children are healthy from the moment you find out they're coming into the world. During pregnancy, your baby is as much a part of you as your internal organs. By eating healthy foods, exercising, and destressing, not only will you feel better physically and emotionally, you'll also create a solid, healthy foundation for both you and your baby.

Women who adopt and maintain healthy lifestyles throughout pregnancy generally have fewer risks and complications, straight-forward births, and an easier time bouncing back postdelivery than those who don't. When I say "healthy lifestyle," I'm talking about balancing the food and supplements you consume, exercising, and managing stress. And this lifestyle doesn't have to end once you give birth—by shifting your habits, you'll feel better for life.

It's never too late—or too early—to establish a healthy routine. During the first month of pregnancy, you may not even realize that you're pregnant, so it makes sense to take stock of your prepregnancy lifestyle. Note the foods you've been eating, whether you're mostly active or sedentary, and how stressed-out you feel on a daily basis. Evaluating your lifestyle now will help you to create a healthy environment for yourself and your children in the future. The better care you take of yourself during pregnancy, the better care you'll be taking of the baby within you. Your baby is dependent on you to make choices that best support her growth and development. Changing less-than-ideal eating and lifestyle habits during the first month of your pregnancy lays the foundation for the months (and years!) to come. This chapter explores why mind/body health matters for you *and* your baby.

"The greatest wealth is health."

—Virgil

YOUR CHANGING BODY

Are you really pregnant for 10 months instead of 9? If you've just found out that you're pregnant, your doctor probably did the math to arrive at a due date 40 weeks away. Caregivers calculate your due date from the beginning of your last menstrual cycle, since it's difficult to pin down the actual date of conception. So for calculation purposes, you're "pregnant" before you even conceive.

The first month of pregnancy is an exciting yet fragile time, one with a lot of questions, concerns, and the beginning of many strange physical and emotional feelings. You may not feel overly sick or tired just yet, but that doesn't mean there aren't major developments going on! Many women experience subtle symptoms of pregnancy in the beginning, while others don't even notice. Early symptoms include:

- Missed period
- Tender breasts and nipples
- Aversions to certain foods or smells
- Mood swings
- Cravings for certain foods
- Tiredness and general fatigue

At this point, there's more happening in your uterus than anywhere else in your body. You may not be feeling any pregnancy "symptoms" by Week Four, but there are lots of ways to connect with yourself and your rapidly growing baby-to-be.

"CALLING IN" YOUR BABY

"The deeper the roots, the higher the branches."
—Unknown

Sit in a comfortable position in a quiet space where you won't be disturbed. Place your hands on your lower belly and begin to breathe in through your nose, feeling your breath in your belly. Do this for 4 slow counts. Exhale for 4 slow counts as you allow your whole belly and body to relax and soften. Do this deep-breathing cycle three times.

Next, imagine a baby—your baby—and slowly begin to deep-breathe again. Breathe in while picturing this baby, again breathing through your nose and into your belly. While you are breathing, visualize becoming pregnant with this child. As you exhale, relax and soften your body, allowing your body to receive this baby. Again, repeat three times.

Begin to see yourself with your baby. Imagine the child and what it would be like for you and your partner to be together with this baby. Envision and, more importantly, *feel* your life with this child. Notice how you feel being her mother, having her in your arms, close to you. Name that feeling (joy, love, bliss, etc.), breathe that feeling into your heart, and exhale anything out that might be blocking you (for example, stress, doubt, or fear). Allow this positive feeling to flood over you as you *let go* of disappointment, sadness, or worries.

See your baby in your arms and from this loving place in your heart talk to her, telepathically or out loud. Tell her (as you feel this energy) how much you can't wait to be her mother; show her what her life with you will be like, let her know you are ready for her to "Come home to me now," that you are open and ready to receive her and can't wait to hold her in your arms. Show her all you have been doing to prepare and ask if she needs anything from you. You might hear something or you might not. Keep talking as long as you need to, and end with "*Come home to me now. I am open and fully ready to receive you into my heart and into my life.*"

Next, cut out inspirational pictures of couples, families, and babies and glue them onto a tall, glass-encased white candle or large piece of paper. Add pictures of yourself, your partner, dog, parents, or perhaps places you love. Place objects that are meaningful to you around the candle or sheet of paper (crystals, goddess statues, baby clothes) like you are making a baby altar.

Place a few drops of scented oil into the top of the candle and light it. Let the candle burn all the way down.

After you do the visualization from the calling-in ritual (above), write a heartfelt letter to your baby. It's never too early to start communicating with your baby, even through words on paper. I also suggest starting a baby book, journal, or scrapbook—something to collect your keepsakes, photos, and memories of meaningful moments of your pregnancy and birth. Start the book with this special letter. This will be something to share with your child as he grows to show how much he was loved before he was born.

Writing a letter to your baby-to-be can be the first connection you make with the tiny person inside you. It doesn't have to be a long letter, just something from your heart that speaks to you and your child about the journey you're both about to embark on. Engage your partner, too, and you'll both have a chance to express your thoughts to your new addition.

WHAT TO EAT FOR THE FIRST MONTH

"Don't eat anything your great-grandmother wouldn't recognize as food."

—Michael Pollan

Food is a major focus during pregnancy. It serves as the basis for your baby's growth and survival. Eating a well-rounded, balanced diet full of organic, hormone-free, genetically modified organism (GMO)–free whole foods is ideal, especially during pregnancy. Each month, as your body and baby grow together, I'm going to highlight specific food groups and types of food to focus on. This doesn't mean you should stop eating other healthy food groups you've already incorporated into your diet. The growing list of foods I will provide offers a wide variety of healthy and tasty options for you during your entire pregnancy.

Did you know that what a woman consumes while pregnant shapes her child's palate later on? Studies from the Monell Chemical Senses Center have shown the food that mom eats flavors the amniotic fluid, which in turn is swallowed by the fetus. Babies are actually "tasting" foods! You have the opportunity to teach your baby to love healthy foods before he's even born (which is a lot easier than teaching a toddler).

There is a common misconception that "eating for two" during pregnancy means you need to consume a lot more food. Not true! While pregnant, you need to consume only 250 more

EATING HEALTHY ON A BUDGET

Eating healthy does not have to mean breaking the bank! Follow these tips for balanced nutrition on a budget.

- Grow your own garden. Even if you can only grow herbs like basil, oregano, and parsley or a few vegetables, you'll save money on seasonings (and your food will taste better than anything packaged).

- Buy foods like beans, grains, nuts, and pastas in bulk. They're less expensive when you buy more at once, and they keep well in a dry pantry for a long time.

- Prioritize what's most important to buy organic. Look at the Environmental Working Group (EWG) Web site, which lists the "Dirty Dozen," the fruits and veggies that absorb the most pesticides and so should be eaten organic.

- Shop at local farmers' markets and buy produce that is in season. These foods tend to be less expensive because they are at their peak of production.

- Buy generics. Stores such as Whole Foods and Trader Joe's have their own brands, which are generally less expensive and taste just as good. Many other grocery stores have their own organic brands, too.

- Eat out less. Browse the cookbook shelf to find recipes that excite you. Turn on some music, set a pretty table, and enjoy the process of cooking and dining at home.

- Plan out your meals for the week ahead before you go food shopping. Make a list and buy only what you plan to prepare for the week. This will cut down on fresh food that spoils before you can use it and impulse buys that you really don't need.

calories per day than before pregnancy. Chances are, if you're eating a typical American diet, you're getting way more than the daily calories you need, even with a growing baby. Instead of worrying about eating *enough* food, focus more on the food's *quality*. The healthier you eat, the better you will feel and the stronger your body will be to support your pregnancy and labor. You can shift your awareness simply by asking yourself these two questions: How is this food feeding me? How is it fueling my baby's development?

Here are my top tips for building a healthy nutritional foundation for you and your baby.

Eat as Organic as You Can

Organic foods are certified to be free of any chemical treatments. Pregnant women and children are the most vulnerable to these toxins. The *Fourth National Report on Human Exposure to Environmental Chemicals* by the Centers for Disease Control (CDC), updated in 2014, measured pesticides and other chemicals in the bodies of Americans every few years. Results of the study consistently show that pesticides cross the placenta and can be absorbed by the fetus during pregnancy.

Growth hormones are found in cattle, poultry, and eggs that don't come from organic farms. Growth hormones have been linked to certain cancers and can alter hormone production, which, according to a study from the Cincinnati Children's Hospital, can lead to early puberty in girls and cause development and reproductive problems. Organic foods might cost a little more, but can you really put a price on your family's health?

Eat for Fuel

Whole foods (nonprocessed, fresh, high-quality, nutrient-rich foods) are filled with a ton of healing properties. Take bananas, for example. These sweet, simple fruits are both high in potassium and rich in iron, which can help your nerves and muscles function properly as well as help carry oxygen throughout your blood. Their serotonin boosts mood, fiber helps battle constipation, and alkaline properties help neutralize stomach acidity from heartburn or ulcers.

When we see how food *really* feeds us, both physically and emotionally, our relationship with food and eating will change. Food truly is fuel to get your body to move, grow, feel, and heal. My intention in teaching you about the healing properties of foods is that when you eat, you'll connect with how this food is doing something not only for your body, but for your baby, as well. After working with me, lots of my clients develop a new relationship with food. I see them eat completely differently than they used to and even feed their children with the intention of doing something positive for their lives.

Increase Your Intake of Vitamins, Minerals, and Supplements

A good prenatal vitamin helps to ensure that you and your growing baby are getting a balanced amount of vitamins and minerals each day. It's best to start taking one a few months before trying to get pregnant, but don't worry if you didn't. However, as soon as you find out you're pregnant, finding a prenatal vitamin is essential. I prefer food-based (nonsynthetic) vitamins, as they're the most natural form and are easier to digest. One prenatal vitamin a day, however, won't give you the extra boost of many vitamins and minerals that will help prep your body and baby for growth. Here are some vitamins and supplements I think are essential to take during pregnancy.

Vitamin D (up to 4,000 IU a day): Most prenatal vitamins contain around 400 IU of vitamin D. A study from *Diabetologia* (the journal of the European Association for the Study of Diabetes) explains that increasing your vitamin D intake up to 4,000 IU a day can reduce your risk of gestational diabetes, preeclampsia (pregnancy-related high blood pressure), and premature birth.

Did you know that vitamin D is known as the "sunshine vitamin"? The body produces it naturally when exposed to sunlight. Believe it or not, an easy way to get extra vitamin D while pregnant is to go outside around noon and sit in the sun with your belly exposed for 10 to 20 minutes. I also like vitamin D drops, especially for those who hate swallowing pills. Place a few drops on your tongue, and you're done for the day.

Vitamin E (400 to 600 IU a day): In the book *For the Childbearing Year*, Susun Weed, an herbalist and director of the Wise Woman Center in Woodstock, New York, explains that taking vitamin E throughout the first trimester helps the embryo adhere to the wall of your uterus and has been shown to help prevent miscarriage. Stop taking vitamin E after the third month to prevent abnormal adhering.

Probiotics: These healthful, "good" bacteria live in your colon. When "bad" bacteria form in your gut, causing diarrhea or a yeast infection, probiotics replenish the good bacteria and help restore your belly's balance. The most popular probiotic is *Lactobacillus acidophilus*, found in yogurt and other cultured

Getting enough water in your system every day is vital for a healthy pregnancy. Water flushes toxins and wastes from your body, which you have more of due to the baby. Water also combats dry, itchy skin, constipation, fatigue, and swelling. Drinking enough water also helps prevent bladder infections, hemorrhoids, preterm labor, preeclampsia, and miscarriage. You can drink water from the tap, of course, but water is also abundant in many fruits and vegetables. The following foods are more than 90 percent water and can help keep you hydrated during the day: cantaloupe, watermelon, pineapple, tomato, blueberries, grapefruit, cucumber, and lettuce.

foods. (Look for the phrase "live and active cultures" on the label.) Probiotics can be found in pill or powder form or in dairy products such as kefir or yogurt, which can be added to smoothies or cereal if you don't like to eat dairy alone.

During pregnancy, probiotics promote gut health and healthy digestion and help prevent constipation and diarrhea by calming and balancing the digestive track. A study published in the journal *Lancet* explains that probiotics may also help prevent food allergies and eczema in young children, as well as prevent urinary tract infections in mom and strengthen the immune system of both mom and baby.

Powdered greens: Add a powdered, mixed-green supplement to your smoothie if you're not a big veggie eater. I love powdered greens and "supergreens," such as spirulina, blue-green algae, and sun chlorella. These plant-based supplements are great to oxygenate your blood and help protect both you and your baby from free radicals and toxins.

I also recommend increasing your intake of the following minerals and nutrients.

Calcium: Calcium isn't only for the development of strong bones and teeth. It can also help with leg cramps and insomnia. You don't have to gulp down multiple glasses of milk to get enough calcium, however. Calcium can be found naturally in many other foods, including dairy products such as cheeses and yogurt; soy products, including soybeans, tofu, and tempeh; tahini, almonds, and almond butter; orange juice; calcium-fortified rice milk, soy milk, or almond milk; calcium-fortified tomato juice; dried figs; broccoli; dark green leafy vegetables such as kale, bok choy, turnip greens, and collard greens; fish such as sardines and salmon; parsley; seaweed; and beans.

Essential fatty acids (EFAs)/omega-3s. These oils are vital for the normal development of the fetal retina, nervous and immune systems, and brain. (Seventy percent of all EFAs go to the brain.) They also help reduce your chances of developing preeclampsia, postpartum depression, and preterm labor.

Here are some foods that contain omegas: oils, such as olive, canola, fish, hempseed, and flaxseed oil; seeds, such as flax, hemp, sesame, pumpkin, sunflower, and chia seeds; nuts, including walnuts, almonds, and nut butters; lentils; split peas; soy products, including tofu and soybeans; wheat germ; fatty fish, including salmon and cod; and veggies, including avocados, kale, spinach, collard greens, and winter squash.

Iron is essential for making hemoglobin (the protein in red blood cells that transports oxygen to other cells). An iron deficiency is called anemia, which is very common in pregnancy. Foods high in iron are liver, meat, poultry, and dark-meat turkey; fish; foods cooked in cast-iron cookware; brewer's yeast; blackstrap molasses; beans, such as soybeans and navy, lima, kidney, black, and pinto beans; lentils and chickpeas; sea vegetables; winter squash; dried fruits such as apricots and raisins; prunes and prune juice; pumpkin seeds; oatmeal; millet; and whole wheat bread.

Protein is the basic building block for all babies' tissues and cells. The growth of the placenta and uterus, the extra blood supply, the making of breast milk, and the structure of the baby's brain are largely dependent on the proteins we consume. Protein is found in meats, poultry, fish, eggs, milk, soybeans, soy products, yogurt, spirulina, cottage cheese, other cheeses, kidney and other beans, lentils, nuts, and seeds.

Antioxidants can be found as vitamins, minerals, or phytochemicals (special plant compounds). They help repair cell damage caused by free radicals, which can attack your immune system. Some researchers also believe that free-radical damage may be involved in promoting chronic diseases such as heart disease and cancer.

If you're thinking about picking up an "antioxidant-rich" vitamin supplement, don't be fooled. Each fruit and veggie has its own unique combination of antioxidants—you won't find any of these specialized combos isolated in a pill. Your best bet is to eat a variety of seasonal produce so you can reap all the benefits. A good trick to remember to get enough antioxidant-rich foods is to "eat the rainbow." Eating a lot of colorful fruits and vegetables is a great way to make sure you are eating foods high in antioxidants.

Folic acid, also called folate, is an important B vitamin that plays a vital role in the early stages of pregnancy. In the beginning of pregnancy, folic acid helps in the production of red blood cells and aids in the development of your baby's neural tube, brain, and spinal cord. Folic acid helps prevent birth defects such as spina bifida and other abnormalities of the spine and brain in the first trimester; low birth weight and miscarriage; and later pregnancy complications such as preeclampsia.

Folic acid is found in every prenatal vitamin available, but it's also found in many natural foods. You may even have been taking folic acid in advance of your pregnancy. (But if you haven't, it's okay.) Here's how much folic acid is recommended, by stage of pregnancy.

- While you're trying to conceive: 400 to 600 micrograms
- For the first 3 months of pregnancy: 400 micrograms
- For the 4th through 9th month of pregnancy: 600 micrograms
- While breastfeeding: 500 micrograms

The National Institute of Neurological Disorders and Stroke (NINDS) recommends taking 400 micrograms, or 0.4 milligram, of folic acid both before conception and during pregnancy to decrease the risk of neural tube defects such as spina bifida by up to 70 percent. Foods high in folic acid include dark green vegetables, egg yolks, and some fruits. Many foods, such as cereals, enriched breads, and pastas and other grains, are now fortified with folic acid. Many multivitamins contain the recommended dosage of folic acid as well.

Now is the perfect time to really evaluate your eating habits and food choices. Ask yourself: How is this food fueling me? How is it feeding my developing baby? Is this the best choice? If the answer is no, ask yourself: What can I eat instead that would benefit us *both*?

A gardener always prepares the soil to be as healthy and nourished as he can *before* planting precious seeds. The healthier the soil, the healthier and more vibrant plants those seeds will grow. Our bodies are like this as well—the healthier your body is during pregnancy, the better the environment for maintaining a healthy pregnancy and supporting a flourishing child.

During the first month of pregnancy, I always recommend my clients eat a well-balanced diet with an emphasis on antioxidant-rich foods and foods high in folic acid. Each day, millions of old cells die and millions of new cells are born. The first few weeks are all about cell division in your developing baby. By focusing on a diet rich in antioxidants and folic acid during Month One, you will better protect the new cells that make up your baby from free radicals, chemicals, pollution, and radiation. And you'll be protecting your own body, too!

Choose foods from the following lists.

FOODS HIGHEST IN ANTIOXIDANTS

- Berries, including blueberries, blackberries, raspberries, acai berries, goji berries, cranberries, and strawberries
- Beans, including kidney beans, red beans, black beans, and pinto beans
- Seeds, including chia seeds and poppy seeds
- Broccoli
- Artichokes
- Dried fruits, including prunes, dates, raisins, and apricots
- Apples, including Red Delicious, Granny Smith, and Gala varieties
- Stone fruits, including peaches, plums, and cherries
- Citrus fruits such as oranges, grapefruits, papayas, and guavas

- Nuts, including pecans, walnuts, and hazelnuts
- Tomatoes
- Dark green leafy vegetables, such as kale and spinach
- Orange foods, including carrots, pumpkin, squash, and sweet potatoes
- Bell peppers of all colors
- Cantaloupe
- Corn
- Dark chocolate and cacao (in moderation, of course!)
- Spices and herbs, including cinnamon, oregano, and fresh parsley
- Decaffeinated green tea
- Fish, such as salmon

FOODS HIGHEST IN FOLIC ACID

- Whole grains and fortified cereals
- Bananas
- Blackberries, strawberries, and blueberries
- Yogurt
- Asparagus, green beans, peas, broccoli, Brussels sprouts, raw spinach, and other dark green leafy vegetables
- Avocados
- Mushrooms
- Orange juice
- Sunflower seeds
- Egg yolks
- Legumes such as lentils, beans, and split peas
- Barley and brown rice

 JOURNAL WORK: STARTING A FOOD LOG

"Your body is a temple, but only if you treat it as one."
—Astrid Alauda

Studies have proven that one of the most effective ways to gauge how healthy you're eating is to write down everything you put in your mouth. Listing the foods you eat and drink, as well as portion sizes, can reveal what you need to change to get the optimal benefits from eating healthy. For your first journal work, I suggest keeping a detailed list of the foods you eat. This will help you clean up and rebalance your diet, and it will put you well on your way to being a healthy mom for your baby.

For 2 weeks, keep as accurate a food log as possible, including drinks, supplements, and snacks. As the days go by, answer as many of the questions below as possible.

- What time did you wake up? How many hours of sleep did you get?

- What supplements are you taking, and what time of the day are you taking them?

- How do you feel upon waking? Are you still tired or are you energized, nauseated or hungry?

- What meals, snacks, and drinks did you have throughout the day, and at what times?

- If you exercised, what activity did you do? For how long?

- What was your stress level for the day? Rate it from 1 to 10, with 1 being low and 10 being very high.

- What time did you go to sleep?

After keeping this food log for 2 weeks, review it. See where you can make some adjustments. Ask yourself:

- Are you getting enough sleep?

- During what part of the day are you the most tired? Do you find that you're tired at the same time every day, or do you feel tired after eating bread or foods that contain sugar?

- How much are you moving your body? Are you moving enough or even too much, and need more rest?

- Are you skipping meals or letting too much time pass before eating again?

- When do you eat—at regular intervals or when you're stressed or emotional?

- Are you drinking enough water?
- Are you eating enough food for the amount of energy you're expending?
- Are you eating whole foods, organic foods, and a variety of colors?

This is the first exercise I perform when working with a new client. You don't need to go crazy and totally alter your diet and lifestyle all at once! I try to tweak habits, perhaps by replacing a food with a better alternative or providing resources about the benefits of sleep and exercise. The ability to see your eating, sleeping, exercising, and stress patterns on paper is a great start. Understanding your habits—both good and bad—is the first step in making any necessary improvements, both for yourself and your baby.

FRUIT AND VEGGIE WASH

How you clean your produce is as important as where your produce came from. Try this simple wash to remove unwanted dirt or gunk from your fruits and veggies.

- Spray bottle (BPA-free plastic or glass)
- 3 tablespoons white vinegar
- 1 cup water
- 1 medium organic lemon, halved

Clean the spray bottle well with warm water. Add the vinegar and water to the bottle. Squeeze in as much juice from the lemon halves as you can. Give the bottle a shake and you're good to go.

MOVE IT! EXERCISE AND PREGNANCY

I'm always telling my clients that keeping active during pregnancy will bring huge advantages to their bodies and babies. Exercise is *so* important. Whether you've been a marathon runner, yoga enthusiast, or someone who barely set foot in a gym before pregnancy, exercise is a positive way to:

- Gain more energy
- Sleep better
- Reduce stress
- Stay regular (ease constipation)
- Lift your spirits (thanks to the endorphins it releases)
- Increase the odds of an easier labor
- Help your body bounce back faster postdelivery
- Reduce the risk of gestational diabetes and high blood pressure during pregnancy

So many questions are associated with exercising while pregnant. Whatever your current fitness level, the best advice I can give you is to listen to your body. Now is the time to honor your body and the baby you're bringing into the world, and exercise is a great way to do that. Don't be afraid to ask your caregiver if you want to make any changes in your exercise routine.

If you're just starting to exercise, start slowly! As you'll see in this book, I'm a big fan of yoga. If you're new to yoga, consider trying a prenatal yoga class designed just for pregnant women. If you've been doing yoga for a while now, keep going to your normal class. Just don't do any poses that involve twisting or crunching your abs, and avoid getting overheated. Your instructor will be able to help modify any poses you're not sure about doing.

Here are some things I talk about with my clients when we start to work out an exercise program for them.

- Listen up! Your body will naturally give you signs that it's time to slow down or stop what you're doing.
- Wear the proper shoes for whatever activity you're doing, such as sneakers with ankle and arch supports.
- Never exercise to the point of exhaustion or breathlessness. This is a sign that your baby and your body cannot get the oxygen supply they need.
- Take breaks if needed, and drink plenty of fluids during exercise.
- Exercise outside as much as you can, but be careful when exercising in extremely hot weather. This can cause dehydration.
- Avoid rocky terrain or unstable ground when running or cycling. Your joints are more lax in pregnancy, and ankle sprains and other injuries may occur.
- Avoid contact sports.
- Lifting weights is okay, as long as you aren't straining your body.
- During the second and third trimesters, avoid exercise that involves lying flat on your back, as this decreases bloodflow to the uterus.
- It's a good habit to include gentle stretching and warmup activities before you exercise, as well as relaxation and a proper cooldown after your workout.
- If you're used to exercise, you can continue to work out at the same level while you're pregnant. Ask your caregiver about limitations to your current exercise routine. Each trimester might bring new physical challenges, so it's important to tune in to your body and tailor your exercise plan to your needs.

Prenatal Yoga

As a pregnancy coach and doula, I provide a healthy and supportive program to help my clients through their entire pregnancies. One thing I encourage all of my clients to try, whether at home or in a class, is prenatal yoga. Yoga is an amazing way to gently stretch the body, promote good circulation, and support natural ways to heal many pregnancy ailments. Yoga helps increase bloodflow throughout the body, and even to the brain. The kind of yoga I teach is gentle, healing, and transformative. I combine restorative and yin yoga with breathwork, chakra movements, and visualizations to help clear the mind, calm the body, and renew and ground energy levels.

These calming and nurturing restorative yoga poses and chakra movements are great to practice daily or as often as time permits during the first few months of pregnancy (or even while trying to conceive). They all increase circulation and nourish the reproductive organs. The more you link your breathing to the specific areas of the body you want to "open up," the more energy you will move. Doing isolated breathwork actually nourishes the area you are breathing into with oxygen, which in turn increases bloodflow. It also helps generate body awareness during pregnancy, connecting you with your baby within you and, later, during birth. You can do just one pose at a time or do the whole sequence. I suggest a few rounds of breathwork for each, but if it feels good and you want to go longer, by all means keep going. A round of these poses takes 10 to 15 minutes total. It's a great way to start or end your day and connect to your body and baby.

RECLINING BOUND ANGLE POSE

This pose is a gentle groin opener.

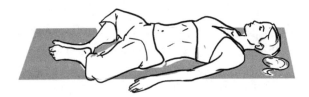

Lie on your back and bend your knees, with your feet flat on the floor as close to you as possible. Bring your feet together and allow your knees to open down toward the floor. Begin to imagine your baby! Let yourself feel the joy and excitement of having this baby, and slowly breathe that vision and feeling in through your nose deep down into your belly. As you exhale slowly, breathe out any worry, stress, or tension through your mouth as you allow your body to relax and open to receive your baby. Do this for 10 breaths or more.

RECLINING PIGEON POSE

Our hips are a dumping ground for repressed emotion. This pose releases emotions and stress while increasing bloodflow and energy to the reproductive organs.

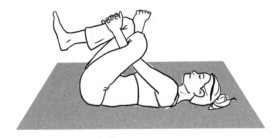

Lie on your back. Bend your knees, and place your feet flat on the floor, hip-distance apart. Cross your right ankle over your left knee and flex your right foot. Place your right arm between your legs and wrap your left arm around your left knee. Slowly bring your knee toward your chest. Inhale slowly through your nose for 4 counts, sending the breath into the tight area of your hip or groin. As you exhale slowly through your mouth for 4 counts, breathe out that tightness and tension as you allow your hips to soften and relax. Do this for 10 breaths and then switch sides.

HIP CIRCLES

This pose increases circulation and bloodflow while loosening up the hip joints and lower back.

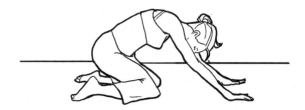

Start the pose on all fours, with your hands flat on the floor under your shoulders and your knees on the floor a little farther than hip-distance apart. Begin to slowly circle your hips to the left, then forward, to the right, and then to the back, making a fluid circle. Close your eyes and put your whole body into it, making it a seductive, sensual movement. The slower you move, the calmer your energy becomes. Circle 10 times starting to the left side, and then circle 10 times starting to the right side.

BUTTERFLY POSE

This pose opens the groin and hips, increases circulation, and stimulates the ovaries.

Begin by sitting on the floor with your spine straight and legs straight out in front of you. Bend your knees, sliding your heels toward your pelvis. Naturally drop your knees out to your sides. Press the soles of your feet together, pushing the outer edges of your feet into the floor as you wrap your hands around your feet or ankles.

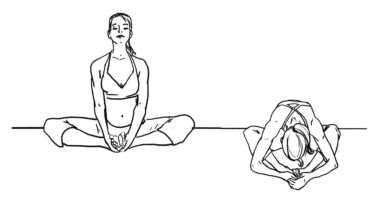

This pose offers a couple of variations. You may choose to stay in this position for the rest of the pose. If you do, keep your spine as straight as you can. Breathe in through your nose for 4 counts while speaking or thinking the word "Let." Then exhale through your mouth slowly for 4 counts while saying or thinking the word "go" as your groin opens and your knees relax closer to the floor. For the variation, inhale through your nose the same as before, and breathe in for 4 counts with the word "Let." Then exhale through your mouth as you fall forward while saying or thinking "go." You should feel your spine lengthening as you bend forward. Breathe for 10 counts.

WIDE-ANGLE SEATED FORWARD BEND

This pose stimulates bloodflow, nourishes the ovaries, and opens the groin.

Sit on the floor with your legs straight out in front of you. Open your legs like a V with your knees facing up to the sky. Raise your arms over your head as you inhale, while stretching your spine. Exhale as

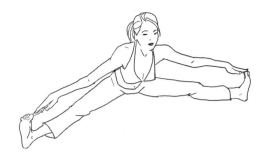

you bend forward (without rounding your back), and place your hands on your ankles or shins. Hold this pose for 1 minute, concentrating your breathing into the groin area. Inhale, thinking about peace and calm, and exhale any tension or tightness through your mouth as your groin area relaxes and softens with each breath.

LEGS ON THE WALL POSE

This pose is a little tricky to get into, but once you get there, it's pure bliss. It not only calms the nervous system, it also nourishes your pelvic region by flooding the whole area with blood and oxygen. While you practice your breathing, the more you can relax and let go when exhaling, the more easily blood can nourish and feed your body. This pose is also great to do after having sex when you're trying to conceive as well as through the first trimester to help prevent miscarriage. It helps with hemorrhoids, swollen legs, and is simply a very comfortable pose to enjoy.

Find a wall space and place a bolster, a few folded blankets, or a couple of pillows a few inches from the wall for support. Lie with your legs up on the wall for 10 minutes, two times a day.

Close your eyes and let your arms fall to your sides. Begin to slowly and deeply breathe in through your nose for 4 counts, sending the breath down into your belly. Begin exhaling slowly through your nose for 4 counts as you allow your whole body to soften and relax. Feel the ground supporting you. Breathe in this affirmation: "I trust the universe has my back. All is unfolding perfectly and as it should be. I trust divine timing. I am exactly where I am meant to be." Now, breathe out the affirmation: "All is well. The universe is working for my highest good." Repeat this breathing actively and consciously 10 times.

A GREENER PREGNANCY

"We do not inherit the earth from our ancestors,
we borrow it from our children."

—Native American proverb

A person can go crazy trying to avoid all the toxins in today's world. Toxins are everywhere—in the air we breathe, food we eat, clothing we wear, water we drink, and even products we use to clean our homes and our bodies. My intention is not to create fear but to raise awareness. We can't change everything surrounding us, but we can be proactive in the choices we make to stay as healthy as possible, especially during pregnancy. The very best place to start making the world healthier and safer is right in your own home.

Eat local and organic. Organic foods are grown without the use of pesticides, synthetic fertilizers, sewage sludge, or GMOs. Organic labels assure you that the animals from which your meat, poultry, eggs, and dairy products come have not been given antibiotics or growth hormones. Always look for the USDA seal to ensure the quality of the organic foods and products you purchase. When you buy your food locally, you get fresher food while also strengthening your local economy, supporting family farms, and reducing carbon dioxide emissions and packaging materials due to long traveling times.

Use nontoxic cleaning supplies. Always look for cleaning supplies labeled "nontoxic" or "ecofriendly" that are biodegradable as well as petroleum, phosphate, volatile organic compound, and solvent free. You can also make your own, and I promise they are simple and cost efficient to make. Later on in this chapter, I'll tell you how to make a few effective and amazing-smelling supplies that aren't toxic for you or your home. You'll never buy another bottle of spray cleaner again!

Stay away from plastic water bottles and containers. If you do use plastic, make sure it's labeled "BPA-free." BPA (bisphenol A) is a chemical found in hard plastics and the coatings inside canned foods and drinks. It mimics estrogen and has been known to disrupt normal hormone levels and development in fetuses and babies. Drinking from glass containers is always better, if it's possible! Also, a better choice than canned foods would be fresh, organic whole foods.

Use organic, fragrance-free skin care products. Be sure the products you buy are labeled "phthalate-free" and "paraben-free." Phthalates are used to soften plastics and make them more flexible to prevent them from becoming brittle and cracking when bent. They are also added to products to help them lubricate and penetrate into the skin. Phthalates and other chemicals can hide behind the word *fragrance,* because they're added to products to help their fragrances last longer. Parabens are preservatives used to prevent bacterial growth in cosmetics amd beauty products. Both phthalates and parabens are hormone disrupters. Instead, organic coconut oil is a great skin moisturizer to use after a shower. I add essential oils to a jar of unscented coconut oil and make a soothing blend of ylang-ylang, orange, and rose. A great resource to see how safe your products are is the Environmental Working Group's Skin Deep Cosmetics database at, ewg.org/skindeep/.

Use plants in your home to naturally filter the air. A beautifully green way to filter the air in your home is with plants. Houseplants filter indoor air by producing oxygen from carbon dioxide. They also absorb the toxic airborne chemicals benzene, formaldehyde, and trichloroethylene, which can be present in house paint, cleaning supplies, and carpeting. Some of the best air-filtering houseplants that would also make your home beautiful are:

- Ivies, including English ivy and devil's ivy
- Spider plants
- Philodendrons, including elephant ear, heartleaf, and selloum

(continued on page 28)

CLEANING UP YOUR CLEANING PRODUCTS

This is a quick shopping list to help you prep your home for greener cleaning. Most of the ingredients are inexpensive and easy to find. Essential oils can be a little costly, so choose one or two that you like. You'll only need a few drops per bottle of cleaner, so a little will go a long way! Here are the basic building blocks for natural cleaners.

- **Baking soda** is a great naturally abrasive ingredient with mild alkaline properties. It's also a natural deodorizer and stain remover, it rinses easily, and it's completely nontoxic (no more worries about kids and pets licking surfaces that you've cleaned).

- **Vinegar** is an all-natural and mild acid. It's also a known disinfectant that can remove stains and sanitize, and it's also completely nontoxic. Use white vinegar because of its clear color and purity.

- **Hydrogen peroxide** isn't just a disinfectant for cuts and scrapes. It's also a nontoxic, natural bleaching agent with stain-removing properties.

- **Essential oils,** including lavender, eucalyptus, and geranium, not only help homemade cleaners smell fresh, but these concentrated plant extracts are also disinfecting.

- **Tea tree oil and grapefruit oil** have known antibacterial properties that also help cut through grease and grime.

- **Liquid Castile soap** (like Dr. Bronner's) is a vegetable-based soap, as opposed to a petroleum-based one, which makes it completely nontoxic. It can be used on your face and body but will also work well as a base when cleaning your home.

- **Kosher salt** can be used as a great scrub when mixed with water to form a paste. It even works on cast iron, which can be tough to clean.
- **Distilled water** has no chemicals or salt dissolved in it, so it's a wonderful cleaning base for electronics screen and glass cleaners.
- **Lemon juice** is a natural disinfectant and stain remover and is wonderful for polishing metal. Lemon juice also cuts grease and leaves a totally fresh scent.
- **Borax,** or sodium borate, is a naturally occurring and ecofriendly substance. It can be used to deodorize, remove stains, make an all-purpose cleaning solution, unclog drains, and more. Even through it's natural, borax can be harmful to pets and children if ingested, so use it carefully.
- **Olive or coconut oil** is wonderful to cook with, but it's also a great base for furniture polish. Create a polish with two parts oil to one part lemon juice or white vinegar, shake, and spray.
- **Club soda,** when used with sea salt, helps clean tough stains from carpets and fabrics. The carbonation of club soda also helps remove rust and urine stains.

No shoes in the house! And wipe your pet's paws. While you're out and about, your shoes are collecting pesticides, heavy metals, and dirt from the outside world. Leave your shoes outside the door so none of them get spread around your floors and deposited into your carpets. Also, get into the habit of cleaning your pets' paws before letting them back in the house. This will also minimize the amount of toxins (and dirt) your furry friends bring into your home.

Borrow and share. Pregnancy lasts for only a short time, but maternity clothes can last a lot longer. Ask friends if you can borrow their hand-me-downs, or head to your local consignment shop for maternity clothes and baby gear. Reusing clothing and certain baby stuff will decrease carbon emissions and conserve environmental resources.

It's super easy to find recipes for household cleaners made from the ingredients discussed on pages 26 and 27. The three recipes here are a simple way to start transforming your home into a clean—and green—place that's safe for everyone in your family.

DIY Citrus Vinegar Cleaner

This is a great, all-purpose cleaner you can use every day on windows, glass, or counters.

Peels from 4 or 5 (or more) citrus fruits (oranges, lemons, or limes, or a combination of all three)

Large glass jar

White vinegar

Spray bottle

Place the peels in the jar.

Fill the jar with vinegar and allow it to sit for 2 weeks (no need to refrigerate).

Remove the peels and dilute the vinegar with water (1 cup of water for every 1 cup of vinegar).

Pour into the spray bottle and use immediately.

You can also mix this with a little Dr. Bronner's Castile soap or baking soda for more cleaning power. Try this same recipe with fresh herbs such as sage or rosemary, which also smell great and have antibacterial properties.

Daily Shower Refresher/Mold-Killing Spray

Who doesn't want a shower stall that smells good and is free of grime? This is a great spray that will disinfect your shower walls and keep your shower smelling fresh.

½ cup witch hazel

1½ cups water

¼ teaspoon dish soap (with no colors or fragrance added)

20 drops essential oil (use an oil that's good for killing germs and disinfecting surfaces, such as lemon, lavender, sage, thyme, or tea tree oil)

Combine the witch hazel, water, dish soap, and oil in a spray bottle. Shake well and spray away!

Homemade Air Freshener

Do you have a home with pets, or is your nose starting to be very sensitive to smells? If so, you may want to leave these homemade air fresheners around your house! With only two natural ingredients, you'll feel great knowing you're not breathing in anything toxic. Here's how to make it.

Baking soda

A container, like a small mason jar

Essential oils you would like to smell around the house

Foil (or a lid you don't mind poking holes in)

Pour the baking soda into the container until it is about one-quarter full.

Add 8 to 10 drops of the essential oils.

Cover with the foil or lid. (You'll need to poke holes in the lid, so if you don't want to ruin the jar lid, use the foil.)

Place the jar on a shelf or counter and enjoy the natural scent.

Shake or stir every once in a while when the smell fades.

GREENER SWAPS

INSTEAD OF . . .	TRY . . .
Processed, canned, or frozen foods	Organic, whole, fresh foods
Plastic bottles	Glass bottles or BPA-free containers
Sodas and soft drinks	Sparkling water with pomegranate or cranberry juice
Artificial sweeteners	Natural sweeteners such as stevia or honey
Traditional cleaning supplies	Nontoxic, natural cleaning supplies
Traditional deodorants, creams, etc.	Organic, paraben-free, and sulfate-free products
Synthetic materials (polyester or rayon)	Cotton (preferably organic)

CHAPTER 2

Month Two

MOTHERING YOURSELF

"Self-love is asking yourself what you need—
every day—and then making sure you receive it."

—Unknown

Chances are, by now you're having some morning sickness, you're beginning to feel extremely tired, and your hormones might be raging out of control. This is a time to tune in to *your* needs, nurture yourself, and honor where you are in life. After all, it's very difficult to care for someone else if you're not caring for yourself first. The beginning of pregnancy is also a good time to get comfortable and better prepared to say no when—or, even better, before—you've reached your limit. This chapter will provide tools, exercises, and suggestions for tuning in to your own changing needs and being gentle with yourself as you prepare to become a mother.

Caring for yourself is like being on an airplane when the flight attendant tells you, "In the event of an emergency, first place the oxygen mask on yourself so that you can better assist others." It's the same for you as a mom-to-be. If you're constantly running around without stopping to take a breath, you'll run yourself into the ground and will become totally depleted and of no use to anyone. The more you can take care of and nurture yourself, the better able you'll be to take care of another.

Hopefully, you've practiced being good to yourself throughout your life already. This may have taken various forms—immersing yourself in a hobby or activity like a sport, yoga, or art class; sitting down on the weekend to read a book or have a movie marathon in your living room; getting a massage or trying the hottest new restaurant. Sure, things may change when it comes to personal needs, but the concept is the same.

Tuning in to your needs and recharging your batteries is a way to mother yourself as well as be a better mother to your child. Parenting yourself involves taking care of *your* needs as well, loving yourself enough to know that you matter, too.

"You must manage yourself before you can lead someone else."
—Zig Ziglar

When your child is hungry, you feed him; when he's tired, you help him transition to sleep; when your child is having a bad day, you comfort him. Creating structure and security in a child's life means creating routines, boundaries, and rituals he can count on for consistency and balance. When a child is sick, you nurture and soothe him; when he's been overstimulated, you provide space to give him quiet time; when he's going through a change or something scares him, you give comfort and extra love and support. This is a no-brainer—this is what mothers do!

But how many of you will actually "parent" yourself? I mean *really* take care of yourself? Yes, children constantly need attention and assistance, but adults are expected to be totally competent all the time. Why is it okay to do all of this for children but not set the same standards for ourselves? Why are adults not as important?

When you parent yourself, you're doing much more than you may think. You're setting an amazing example for your children that you care for yourself, which is an act of self-love. There is a saying: "You can't truly love another until you truly love yourself." The same goes for parenting—how can you really be there for another if you can't be there for yourself? The more you show up for yourself, the more naturally and organically you will be able to parent your child. Parenting will become second nature because it will be such a part of you.

During pregnancy, your body is using a tremendous amount of energy to create and house a baby. You can't create or feed a life if you have nothing left to give. This baby you're carrying is feeding off your life force. Pregnancy is a great time to really honor yourself and surrender to your needs. When your baby is born, you'll go into what I like to call the "baby bubble." Many new moms forget about themselves and will naturally put the needs of their babies before their own needs. During pregnancy, you can practice caring for yourself so you'll know when to step back and recharge after the baby comes.

I've worked with a lot of women who say they feel guilty for taking time for themselves, that it's selfish, or that they could be doing something else more "productive" with that time. What's more productive than recharging in order to run more efficiently and happily? I'm here to say that taking a relaxing bath, curling up with a juicy novel, or dedicating time for a massage or yoga practice is *very* productive—not to mention fulfilling. This precious time can generate such positive emotions if you allow yourself the space to experience them. You'll have more patience, be more present and happier, and feel more at peace.

YOUR CHANGING BODY

It only takes a few weeks, and by Month Two you're in the full swing of pregnancy. That swing may, unfortunately, come with a lot of nausea, vomiting, and general hormone increases that can be unpleasant. Your uterus is expanding and is now about the size of a pear, and you're certainly feeling the side effects of starting to grow a person in there. Some symptoms that may have come on suddenly or gradually include:

- Morning sickness and general nausea and/or vomiting
- Increased urination
- Increased fatigue
- Mood swings
- Vivid dreams
- Insomnia
- Sore breasts
- Increased vaginal discharge
- Food aversions and/or cravings

Your body is changing rapidly during this month, even if you don't see many physical changes. You may not have even known you were pregnant until you experienced some of the above symptoms. Often, women don't know there's a baby on the way until a missed period and a general "funny" feeling (especially if this is their first time getting pregnant). Here's why you may be feeling some of the symptoms I've listed above.

Your body's blood production is steadily increasing, to allow for a more rapidly developing baby and expanding belly. The second and third months of pregnancy mark the highest total increase in blood production. Think of the process: Your body produces more blood, your veins have to expand to accommodate the faster-flowing blood, and your heart has to pump faster to allow the blood to support you and reach your baby. You're a well-oiled machine, but the higher circulation demands may be met with protests from the rest of you, which is why you may be dizzy or light-headed.

Hormone production is off the charts! You likely aren't used to so much estrogen, progesterone, and other hormones wreaking havoc on your body—and on your emotions. Those mood swings may be new for you, and they may happen more than you would like. You might not be able to control your emotions, but simply being aware of how you're feeling can help you let it go.

YOUR GROWING BABY

At the beginning of your second month, your baby barely resembles a person and is about the size of an apple seed. By the eighth week, however, the little guy or girl will be about the size of a blueberry and will weigh about a quarter of an ounce. It's hard to think of something as small as an embryo doubling or tripling in size, but that's exactly what your baby is going through right now.

Weeks Five through Eight of a fetus's life concentrate on internal organ development, including the heart, brain, lungs, and intestines. He is growing from a bundle of cells into a small, curved being, ending the month looking more distinct (but still tiny!). Arm and leg buds will begin to appear and the baby's neural tubes—what will form the connections between the brain, spinal cord, and major nerves—will also start to be established.

The second month is also the time baby's face and extremities will start to form. He will have the beginnings of eyelids, ears, a nose, and a chin. He may even be using his webbed fingers and toes to start exploring his surroundings. Of course, you won't feel a thing from the baby just yet. There's still plenty of time to experience the kicks and pushes to let you know your baby is growing and moving.

The surge of progesterone, mixed with high emotions caused by being pregnant, can cause more intense and stranger dreams than usual. And you may remember more of your dreams if you're waking up at night, interrupting phases of dream-filled rapid-eye-movement (REM) sleep.

NAUSEA AND FATIGUE

Nausea, or "morning sickness," is very real for some women and a minor nuisance for others. I'll discuss relief for nausea later in the chapter, but unfortunately, you may just have to ride it out. Thankfully, most of these symptoms often pass in a few weeks. Taking it easy may not be easy at all, but remember, you're honoring your baby by honoring your body. However, if you experience uncontrollable morning sickness, speak with your caregiver about treatment.

Fatigue is almost guaranteed to affect you at different points in your pregnancy. In the beginning, fatigue is a result of the influx of hormones suddenly rushing through your body. Many women are extremely tired during the first couple of months but feel better by the second trimester. By the third trimester, however, weight gain, general aches and pains, frequent trips to the bathroom, and the baby's increased movement bring less sleep.

Alfalfa is a little-known plant that helps with *everything* during pregnancy! Start with one tablet a day and gradually increase to the recommended dose on the bottle. You can find alfalfa tablets at your local health food market or online. Take less if your stools become loose and don't take any at all if you're on blood thinners, since alfalfa is high in vitamin K (a natural blood thickener). Try alfalfa to:

- Ease morning sickness
- Ease heartburn
- Help with constipation
- Reduce anemia
- Reduce postpartum bleeding
- Increase breast milk

Decreased sleep creates a cycle of restlessness and irritability, which in turn brings more stress and anxiety. In Chapter 4, I'm going to talk about how stress can cause problems for your pregnancy and your baby, both in the womb and after birth. I know that beating fatigue while pregnant can be difficult, but to avoid stress (for yourself and your baby), take the time to rest whenever you can. Other ways to fight fatigue include the following:

- Take a B-complex vitamin. This is really helpful in the beginning of your pregnancy. (If taking pills makes you nauseous, try taking a chewable B-complex vitamin.)

- Avoid sugar.

- Avoid caffeine.

- Eat lots of fresh fruits, vegetables, and high-protein foods.

- Cut down on excessive carbs and avoid foods that contain empty calories, such as pretzels, chips, baked goods, etc.

- Meditate, do breathwork, and practice yoga.

- Exercise, even if it's low impact, like walking or swimming.

- Nap when you can.

- Don't be afraid to ask for help! If you can, get help with errands, food shopping, or chores around the house, even if it's for just one task, like laundry or vacuuming. Doing less physical work will ease fatigue and allow for more rest for you and your baby-to-be.

CLIMATE CONTROL

Pregnant women tend to "run hot" and have a difficult time regulating their body temperature. At 99.5°F, your amniotic fluid is slightly warmer than your normal body temperature, to keep your unborn baby warm while she's building up fat stores. This may be why it's the middle of winter yet you're sweating bullets!

Not every pregnant woman experiences sweating, but if you do, it can be annoying. The excess of hormones in your body, an increase in bloodflow to your skin, combined with a higher metabolism that's supporting both you and your baby can lead to a watershed of discomfort. Mild sweating can occur during the day and more excessive sweating at night (called "night sweats").

You won't be able to stop sweating completely, although it may be worse in the beginning of your pregnancy, when your body is first ramping up for pregnancy. Some tricks for staying cool include the following:

- **Dress lightly.** Obviously, if it's freezing outside you don't want to dress for summer. However, layering your clothes will allow you to take off what you need to when you're inside, helping your skin get some air. Wearing next to nothing in the privacy of your own home is your own personal choice, but it *will* bring relief. You can also try wearing organic cotton or other fabrics that wick moisture away, keeping skin cooler.

- **Drink water.** Staying hydrated is something I recommend to my clients anyway, but getting in eight glasses or more of water a day can also help regulate sweating.

- **Cool off with water.** You may already be taking warm baths for relaxation, but a cooler bath will help lower your body temperature (slightly) for a little while. Peppermint oil also has a cooling effect, so add one or two drops (no more than that!) to the water. I once put about 20 drops of peppermint oil into a bath and ended up wearing many layers of clothes and shivering in a ball for 2 hours afterward to warm up! You can also place ice in a damp, wrung-out washcloth and add a drop of peppermint oil to the cloth.

- **Use powder.** Powder will help your skin stay dry and head off uncomfortable heat rash in those out-of-the-way places like behind your knees and between your thighs. Avoid using powders that contain talc, however. Talc is thought to contain traces of asbestos and is not safe to put on your skin or breathe in. There are talc-free powders on the market (try your neighborhood health food market).

Avoid the heat. At one point in your pregnancy, it's going to be summer. Even if you're in the first trimester of pregnancy during the end of the summer season, hot days and sweating go hand in hand. Try to avoid being outside during the hottest part of the day.

Jump in! Getting into a pool can both cool you off and alleviate the pull of gravity on your belly and legs.

I can't stress enough the importance of keeping hydrated. Drinking water won't just cool your body down, like I talked about in Chapter 1, water also removes toxins from your body, keeping swelling down and constipation away. A good rule is to drink one 12-ounce glass every hour throughout the day. Also, you might try drinking alkaline water with a higher pH (such as Qure) for better absorption. You can also add fresh citrus juice to your water to up the alkalinity.

Some tricks to make the water a bit more interesting:

- Make pomegranate juice ice cubes, and add them to your water.

- Water with fresh lemon, fresh mint leaves, and cucumber slices is my summer favorite. The combination is light and refreshing without being too sweet. Muddle the mint at the bottom of a glass to release its oils before adding water.

- Add fresh-squeezed grapefruit, lemon, or orange juice to your water. Putting citrus slices in your glass will also flavor your water nicely.

- Float fresh strawberries, blueberries, or other berries in your water. You can also freeze them into ice cubes and add them to plain water.

- **Use towels at bedtime.** If night sweats are an issue, lay towels on your bed and on your pillow. The towels will absorb sweat better than sheets do and may help you feel a little less like you woke up in a puddle.

- **Sleep cool.** Use a fan, air-conditioning, or open windows to allow extra air to reach you. Try to sleep in light clothing or use light blankets to help keep your body temperature lower at night.

- **Get your thyroid checked.** Your thyroid produces the hormones thyroxine and triiodothyronine, which help regulate metabolism and temperature in the body. Pregnant women often experience a wacky thyroid. A simple thyroid test performed by your doctor can tell if these hormone levels are off. If you're having trouble regulating your temperature, try some of the flavored water mixes discussed on page 39. My favorite is combining watermelon and mint with coconut water. It's healthy, hydrating, and will keep you cool.

It's very common for a partner to gain weight, have morning sickness symptoms, and even feel cramps in his lower abdomen. The condition is known as a "sympathetic pregnancy." This is a perfectly natural response from your partner when faced with both stress and empathy caused by seeing you go through the pregnancy process. Stress releases chemicals in the body that can mimic pregnancy symptoms. And with financial worries, health concerns, and fear of the unknown, pregnancy is often stressful for both parties. Add a little empathy to the mix, and you have a perfect recipe for a sympathetic pregnancy. By keeping your partner involved in your physical and emotional changes, he can share your experience and become more of a partner in the process.

KNOW YOUR LIMITS
AND SET BOUNDARIES

"When you are saying 'yes' to others, make sure you are not saying 'no' to yourself."

—Paulo Coelho

How comfortable are you saying no to people? If that question makes you nervous, read this section carefully. Many women feel the need to say yes or help whenever asked, often at their own expense. Saying no to people or situations can be challenging. You don't want to disappoint someone or seem unwilling to help. But when you constantly say yes—even if your whole being is screaming no—you'll only end up feeling exhausted, aggravated, angry, and overburdened.

Learning to set healthy boundaries with those around you will help ensure healthier relationships, more energy, and a happier life in general. Healthy boundaries will also help you down the road when it comes time to set them for your children. You can only set healthy boundaries (personal rules about or limitations on what you will or can do that suit your own comfort level) by practicing self-awareness of your limits and making self-care your priority. Know that when you care for yourself by setting a rule or limit, you'll have more energy, a more positive outlook, and a better ability to be present for others.

We all have different ways of coping and different limits to what we can (or can't) handle. It's really important to take a good look at how you handle stress and to be truthful about it. It's also important to know why we do the things we do. I need a few hours a day for myself, especially in the morning, to recharge, work out, and write. I also need at least one full day a week off work.

Often, a client will call me at a time I've set aside for myself, and I'll spend an hour helping her. I then get aggravated at myself for not sticking to my work boundaries and end up frustrated because I didn't get to exercise or finish a project or some writing. Why did I do that? (Because I wanted to be accommodating and supportive.) Could it have waited? (Probably.) I could have answered the same questions later, at a better time, without getting frustrated at myself. Instead of giving my time and energy away for free, I could have set up an appointment for a later time, when I was in work mode. So I've set some boundaries for myself professionally: I don't see clients until after noon and I take Saturdays off (unless there's a baby on its way, of course).

KNOW YOUR EMOTIONAL ALARMS

It happens to all of us—we get overworked, stretched to the limit, or we just plain hit a wall. What happens to your emotions when you reach this point? It's different for everyone. I've worked with women who become very aggressive when they're overwhelmed, while some completely go the opposite way—they go numb, shut down, and can't (or don't want to) handle anything. Personally, I get impatient and irritable. I call this an "emotional alarm," and it goes off like a buzzer when we aren't taking enough time to take a break, breathe, and recharge.

Can you think of a time when you were super busy and didn't have the time to recharge your batteries or didn't make enough space in your life for "you" time? How did that make you feel? Also, just as important, how did you treat others when you were feeling this way? This is your trigger emotion, the point where you need some TLC and self-repair.

What do you think your emotional alarms are? By recognizing your alarms early, you can begin to quickly move away from negative reactions and instead be productive with your feelings. By counteracting the energy that comes with being overwhelmed, you'll benefit yourself, your baby, and those around you. This is a good time to make a list of emotional alarms. Fill in the blank in the following sentence.

When I don't get what I need, I am: _____

_____

_____

_____

_____

Identifying an emotional alarm leads to a better set of questions.

- What are your limits when it comes to working with others/ making plans/dealing with family or friends?
- How do you set rules or boundaries?
- Does that mean not doing work before a certain time or turning off your phone in the evening?
- What feelings are triggered when your boundaries have been weakened or you've allowed someone to cross them?

When you feel like a boundary has been crossed, ask yourself:

- How did that happen?
- Could you have shifted the boundary to help yourself? If so, what can you do differently next time?
- How can you be better prepared? Remember my example on page 42.

You might feel guilty telling a friend or family member no when the time comes, or you may worry that the other person might not rely on you anymore. As with anything new or unfamiliar, if you keep practicing enough over time, it will get easier. You'll start feeling so much more confident about your decisions that when other people's feathers get all ruffled because you aren't acting the way they want you to, it won't affect you as much.

Here are some tricks to help you begin setting healthy boundaries with others.

- **Decide what you need or want.** You may need to set different boundaries with different people. Do you need someone to give you more space or respect your time? Take some time to make a list to help pinpoint your needs, so you can move on to the next step. Try starting the list with "I am upset and off-balance with . . ." and take it from there.

- **Be firm.** After deciding what you want, set the boundary. Let's say you're at work and a friend or family member calls you every day, knowing it's inconvenient—and unprofessional—to take personal phone calls. The next time she calls, be very firm and say something like, "I can't take your calls anymore while I'm at work, so please wait until after the workday to get in touch with me." This is an example of a good boundary. You've expressed your feelings respectfully, and you've said what you will no longer do.

When setting boundaries, less is definitely more. You don't need to explain why or how you're setting a boundary, just get right to the point. Clear-cut boundaries leave no room for negotiation or confusion.

- **You're not responsible for the other person's response.** These new boundaries are for you and only you. When you set boundaries, other people might get upset. A good thing to remember is that you have no control over how people will react. All you can really control is the way you choose to show up and handle the situation. Hopefully, in time, the people you've set boundaries with will understand and respect your needs. If you feel guilty about setting a boundary, this is a great opportunity to do some inner work and healing by seeking counseling to help find and clear away the root of this feeling.

- **It's a process!** If you've spent years developing unhealthy boundaries, keep in mind that the changes you're making won't be truly effective overnight. Change takes time, consistency, and practice. It's a process that requires work and willingness to learn and grow. Now that you know you need to value your own feelings as well, setting boundaries can become a productive and successful process.

MORNING AND EVENING TRANSITIONS

One night, after watching an emotional movie and eating pizza, I read an upsetting e-mail from a friend. I had opened the e-mail right before I went to sleep. Already feeling anxious from the movie, I found the e-mail brought up even more emotions. I took that energy to sleep with me that night. I tossed and turned, fell in and out of sleep, and had nightmares. I woke up feeling totally unrested and aggravated. A few minutes after waking up, I checked my phone to find yet another e-mail that intensified all the feelings I had gone to bed with. It took me until the middle of the afternoon to shake off and let go of the negative energy.

The moral of the story? The energy you bring to bed directly affects your sleep, and the energy you wake up with will have a direct effect on your day. I've been talking about honoring your body and mothering yourself as much as you can. What better way to take care of yourself than through a good night's sleep? You need sleep to relax and recharge, but it's difficult to do this effectively when you're going to bed with fear, negativity, and anger. This energy gets embedded in your subconscious and becomes part of your energy field.

Think about the way mothers, fathers, or caregivers transition a child to sleep. They slowly *ease* the child into it. When kids go to bed it's a process, usually some kind of consistent bedtime ritual. They might get a bath, put on pajamas, and go into their room with soft music or nature sounds playing. This peaceful atmosphere leads to a final evening nursing or bottle, a book or two, then goodnight hugs and kisses and wishes for sweet dreams. Parents also tend to know what *not* to give a child before bed. For example, sugar or a large meal will lead to a hyperactive kid, and watching a scary movie before bedtime can cause nightmares.

A teacher of mine once told me, "Whatever we do an hour before bed stays in our subconscious and goes to sleep with us." Just like that, I did away with e-mail, movies, and pizza and replaced them with chamomile tea and a good book. I also start my day by drinking a cup of coffee, lighting candles, listening to classical music, and reading something healing or inspirational.

(continued on page 48)

JOURNAL WORK: PARENTING YOURSELF Q&A

"The greatest gift to others is to freely relinquish yourself."
—Bodhidharma

You may think you know how to best take care of yourself. After all, you've been an adult for a while! You may take pride in your unique personal style, your amazing cooking skills, or the success you've worked hard for in your career. I discussed trigger emotions earlier—the feelings that arise right before you go off the deep end. These triggers are your reminders that it's time to stop and take a breather. Remember, you're important and deserve to be taken care of. You'll not only feel better, but you'll also be a more present and patient parent to your child. Listen to what your body, your mind, and your spirit are telling you—that you need to take action for yourself. Before you begin parenting yourself, here are a few things to ponder.

- Review your lists identifying your trigger emotions and boundary limits.
- If you're feeling tired: What can you do for yourself to regain your energy?
- If you're feeling like you have given too much of yourself: What boundaries have been crossed and how can you better establish new ones?
- If you're feeling sad: What gives you joy?
- What nurtures you or makes you happy?
- What does your spirit need right now?

Put yourself in a child's shoes. Think to yourself, "If this were happening right now to my child, how would I be there for her?" Or, "If my child felt like this, what would I say or do?" As a parent, we will do for our children but not for ourselves. Start turning the tables and applying the ways you would be there for them to be there for yourself. Here are a few examples.

- If you had a child who was upset about something, how would you be there for him? If something upset you, how could you be there and comfort yourself in a similar, loving way?

- If your child were sick, how would you be there for her? If you got sick, what could you do to nurture and care for yourself?

- If your child couldn't sleep because something was bothering him, what would you do? If you can't sleep, what can you do to soothe yourself?

- If your child were tired, what would you do? If you're tired, what can you do to honor that feeling?

If you're feeling drained or overwhelmed and you're not sure how to recharge, here's a simple way to get back on track. Make what I call a "joy list." Write down exercises, activities, hobbies, etc., that nurture and help replenish you, both physically and emotionally. It can be anything—don't be afraid to extend the list onto a new piece of paper! I keep my joy list on my phone and it is filled with activities, people I love, music that helps me focus—whatever nurtures me and gives me joy. Some things on my joy list are yoga, taking my dogs on a hike, dinner with a fun group of friends, getting a massage, or buying fresh flowers.

When you're feeling depleted or tapped out, stop, get your list, pick something, and go do it to recharge your batteries so you can come back fresh and renewed. You, your partner, and especially your baby will thank you! Pregnancy helps you begin to question so many things, and one of them is how to reach your own level of optimal health, both during pregnancy and beyond.

Take these lists and put them up on your fridge, mirror, or somewhere else you can see them easily. Instead of waiting until you're frustrated or tapped out, try to choose something from this list at least two or three times a week and make sure you take the time to complete the activity. It can be as simple as reading one page of an inspirational book or meditating for 5 minutes. Carving out a little bit of time a few days a week to do something special for yourself will give you the confidence, strength, and stamina to be the supermama you are.

If watching the news before bed is your nightly ritual, then think about this: The news is filled with negativity and does nothing but create fear and anxiety. The same goes for having an argument right before you go to sleep. You bring that energy with you into your bed and your subconscious, creating an environment of flux that stays in your mind and body all night. Create a positive ritual for yourself before going to sleep and after first waking up. Try to allow a minimum of 20 to 60 minutes to gently transition into your day in the morning or unwind at night. Remember, how you go to sleep affects your sleep and how you start your day has an effect on the energy of the day.

BREATHWORK FOR RELAXATION

When we are stressed, we naturally hold our breath or we take shallow breaths. Breathing deeply is the fastest way to stimulate the parasympathetic nervous system (relaxation response). Deep breathing is often used to treat anxiety disorders and sleep problems. It releases endorphins, lowers blood pressure, and promotes energy. Deep slow breathing that focuses and directs the breath to a certain body part will help flood that area with oxygen and blood. The slower and deeper you breathe, the calmer and more relaxed you will become. If at any time you are feeling stressed out or anxious, practice a few rounds of breathwork to increase your energy in a snap.

Start with a 5-minute practice, working your way up to 10 to 20 minutes for optimal relaxation benefits. First, breathe normally. Next, close your eyes and scan your body for any tightness. Inhale slowly and deeply through your nose, right into that tight area of your body. Allow your chest and lower belly to rise as you fill your lungs with air. Exhale slowly through your mouth while expelling any tension from your body through your breath as you allow that body part (as well as the rest of you) to soften and relax.

At night, before bed:

- Read something uplifting or positive and inspiring.

- Watch something cheerful.

- Listen to calming or relaxing music or nature sounds.

- Take a hot bath with soothing bath salts (lavender, chamomile, orange, rose, or jasmine) or a long shower; gently scrub your skin with sea salt to remove any negative energy.

- Write your worries and thoughts down on paper. (Putting them in writing will get them out of your mind so you can see that they're not as big a problem as you are making them out to be in your head.)

- Drink warm milk or chamomile tea.

- Meditate.

- Say five things you were grateful for today or in your life.

In the morning:

- Wash with peppermint soap to wake up your senses naturally.

- Do breathwork (breathe in the positive and breathe out the negative). For example, breathe in peace through your nose and breathe out stress through your mouth. Keep breathing in what you need and breathing out what you don't.

- Start the day off by reading a chapter in an inspirational book or a positive affirmation or quote.

- Meditate or chant for 15 to 30 minutes.

- Write in your journal, especially if you recall a dream you had during the night.

- Go for a walk in nature.

- Give yourself a few extra minutes in the morning to exercise or do yoga.

- Return e-mails or read the newspaper over hot tea or coffee.

Try to start putting yourself to sleep like you would a child, in a slow transition filled with nurturing and love. I am not telling you to stop watching the news—just stop watching it right before you go to sleep. Whatever you do to create a nighttime and morning ritual is totally fine. We are all unique individuals with different needs, so make it your own to fit your life. Notice how much better you sleep and how much calmer your day will flow when you start to follow your own, personalized bedtime and morning routines.

HEALTHY COMFORT FOODS

Weeks Six through Ten are the time that I like to call the "foundation of formation" for your baby. It's a time to be mindful of how you're treating your body, including how you eat, move, and rest. During this time, I recommend eating a diet rich in . . . everything! I already spoke about eating the rainbow—foods of every color. In addition, I recommend incorporating the foods in Chapter 1, depending on what you are in the mood to eat. During the second month of pregnancy, when you may feel queasy and tired, I also recommend eating whatever you can get down. Just make sure it's the healthiest choice you can make. You'll get your appetite back soon and be on track to a fulfilling eating experience again.

Are you having cravings yet? You may be looking to go back to the comfort foods of your youth, like macaroni and cheese, pizza, or french fries. It's okay to splurge once in a while. But foods like this can also come back onto your plate in a modern, healthier way. By substituting healthier ingredients, adding veggies, or changing the way you cook something, you can enjoy your favorite comfort foods while still nourishing both you and your baby.

My Healthier Mac and Cheese

1 pound brown rice pasta

3 cups organic whole milk or almond milk

1 cup packed fresh spinach

2 tablespoons organic ghee made with milk from grass-fed cows

2 cups shredded organic Monterey Jack cheese

1 cup shredded organic Cheddar cheese

3 cups chopped broccoli florets

Preheat the oven to 350°F. Coat a 2-quart casserole dish with non-stick spray.

In a large pot, cook the pasta according to package directions, but using a little less salt, until al dente. Reserve ½ cup of the pasta water and strain.

While the pasta is cooking, place the milk and spinach in a blender and blend on high speed until smooth.

In a large pot, melt the ghee. Slowly whisk in the milk mixture and bring to a boil.

Reduce the heat and simmer, whisking occasionally, for 3 to 4 minutes, or until the sauce is gently bubbling.

Add the reserved pasta water and cheeses and whisk until melted. Stir in the pasta and broccoli.

Transfer to the casserole dish. Bake for 30 minutes, or until the cheese is bubbling and the pasta is set.

According to the American College of Obstetricians and Gynecologists, approximately 70 percent of expectant mothers report experiencing some symptoms of morning sickness during the first trimester of pregnancy.

LORI'S MORNING SICKNESS JUICE

This juice is mild in taste and can be sipped throughout the day. Ginger is a great natural remedy for nausea.

3 organic apples

¼"–½" piece organic ginger

3 ribs organic celery

Juice of ½ lemon

Cut the apples into quarters and peel the ginger. Place the apples, ginger, and celery in a juicer. Squeeze in the lemon. Juice together and enjoy cold or at room temperature. Do this every morning for fresh juice that will feed your body and help with the early stages of morning sickness.

NATURAL REMEDIES FOR FIRST-TRIMESTER NAUSEA, MORNING SICKNESS, AND FATIGUE

Morning sickness is caused by hormonal changes, vitamin deficiency, low blood sugar, strong smells and foul odors, lack of exercise, fatigue, stress, constipation, and general anxiety. Morning sickness is more common with the first child if it's a girl or if you are carrying multiple babies, and it is usually the worst between the sixth and twelfth week of pregnancy. Remember, it will be different for every woman and every pregnancy you go through.

Here are some simple, natural remedies to help alleviate morning sickness. Of course, if your morning sickness gets worse, call your caregiver. There are safe medications to relieve morning sickness if you have an extreme case.

❧ Stay hydrated. If water won't stay down, try frozen natural juice popsicles.

- Taking vitamin B$_6$ (25 milligrams) every 8 hours has been shown to have a significant effect in reducing or stopping nausea and vomiting.

- Increase your B-complex and iron intake by taking a food-based B-complex vitamin and iron supplement. Food-based vitamins are nonconstipating and are generally safe to take throughout your entire pregnancy.

- Try zinc supplements (25 milligrams per day).

- Brewer's yeast is high in B vitamins, which prevent nausea. It's good when sprinkled on cereal or rice.

- Drink raspberry leaf, peppermint, or anise tea (all fine during pregnancy).

- Ginger is great in many forms. Fresh ginger can be cut or grated into plain hot water or tea. You can also take ginger in capsule form, drink ginger ale or ginger brew (a healthier choice), or eat ginger chews (candy).

MORNING SICKNESS RELIEF: LEMON ICE CUBES

Many of my clients have morning sickness and tell me this remedy has helped them the most. Lemons have a calming effect on the body and have been known to help relieve nausea.

1 quart water

Juice of 2–4 organic lemons, depending on preferred tartness

Stevia to taste (if you want sweetness)

In a large pitcher or bowl, mix together the water, juice, and stevia (if using). Pour the mixture into an ice cube tray and place it in the freezer at least overnight. Suck on the cubes or crush them and eat them throughout the day.

- Try nux vomica 6x or ipecac 30x, both homeopathic remedies.

- Dilute a few drops of peppermint or chamomile oil in 1 ounce of a base oil, such as olive or coconut oil. Put the mixture on a warm towel and place it over or rub it on your belly.

- Eat a protein-rich snack before bed, such as natural cheese or yogurt.

- Walk or do other mild exercise to relieve hormonal activity.

- Keep a box of crackers by your bed and eat a few before getting out of bed in the morning.

- Avoid spicy, fried, rich, fatty, and greasy foods.

- Avoid any caffeine or artificial sweeteners.

- Get out of bed slowly and avoid sudden movements.

- Get plenty of fresh air.

- Place one drop of peppermint oil on a sugar cube and suck on it.

- Keep apple juice by your bed and sip it through the night (to help keep your blood sugar stable).

- Wear a motion sickness wristband.

- Place two Rescue Remedy drops under your tongue. Rescue Remedy can be found in a yellow Bach Flower remedy bottle.

- Eat five to six small meals a day, so you are eating every few hours. Make sure they have some carbs and some protein to maintain your blood sugar level.

- Try to get a lot of rest; being overtired makes morning sickness worse.

- Try acupuncture. These treatments have been really helpful in treating a few of my clients' morning sickness.

- Avoid strong odors.

Yoga Poses for Morning Sickness

I've been talking a lot about mothering yourself and taking better care of your body. Physically, this can be a tough month for many moms-to-be. You may be extremely nauseous and exhausted and feel generally rundown. This is all a normal part of pregnancy and it will pass! The yoga poses in this chapter can help you with morning sickness and nausea, and they can be done every day, at any time. I promise, they are gentle and easy to do.

SEATED CROSS-LEGGED FORWARD BEND ON CHAIR

Forward bends are great for relaxing and calming. You'll need a chair and one or two pillows.

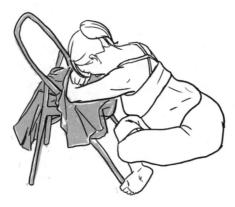

Sit on the floor in a simple cross-legged position with the chair facing you. Place a pillow (or two) on the seat of the chair. Bend your upper body forward and rest your arms on the pillow. Relax your head on your arms and hold for a few minutes. Close your eyes and breathe through your nose deep into your belly. Exhale while allowing your belly to relax and soften.

RECLINING HERO POSE

This pose lifts the diaphragm off the stomach. You will need a yoga bolster or two firm, stacked pillows for support.

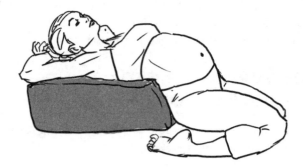

First, come into a kneeling position with your knees hip-distance apart. Slowly lower your bottom to the floor between your heels. Lower your upper body to the floor and bring your arms overhead. Stay in this pose for 1 to 3 minutes.

Make sure to use your arms, not your belly, to push yourself up when coming out of this pose.

Come into Child's Pose for a few seconds or minutes (see Chapter 4 for an explanation and illustration of Child's Pose). Place the pillows or bolster under you for support.

RECLINING BOUND-ANGLE POSE

This pose helps calm and relieve stress, helps with nausea, and opens up the front of the body to relaxation.

You will need a bolster or two firm pillows and a yoga block or four hardcover books for support.

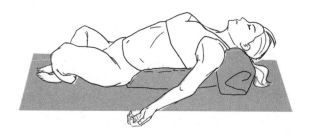

Place a yoga block or stack of books lengthwise under the top end of a bolster or stack of pillows to prop it up on an incline. Sit with your back against the low end of the bolster. Bend your knees with your feet together on the floor and slowly let your legs fall open to the floor, pressing the soles of your feet together. Let your arms fall out to the sides as your chest opens and heart area softens.

BODY SCAN—TUNING IN TO YOUR NEEDS

"It all begins with you. If you do not care for yourself, you will not be strong enough to take care of anything in life."

—Leon Brown

How well do you know your body? What does it need to help you feel relaxed, healthy, and satisfied? Practice this activity regularly to check in with your body and your needs. You can either print out this exercise and do it as part of your daily journaling or close your eyes and make it a visualization exercise. Remember: Don't overthink your answers. Feel your body and go with whatever pops into your head, even if it sounds crazy.

I FEEL	THEY ARE	I NEED
MY FEET		
MY ANKLES		
MY CALVES		
MY KNEES		
MY LEGS		
MY BUTTOCKS		
MY HIPS		
MY GROIN		
MY BELLY		
MY LOWER BACK		
MY MIDBACK		
MY CHEST		
MY SHOULDERS		
MY ARMS		
MY HANDS		
MY NECK		
MY FACE		
MY HEAD		

Notice what comes up over and over for you. What message did you keep hearing? What can you do to support your needs? After you've established where you are and what you need for your body, begin to honor yourself. Here's what I mean: If the words *tired* or *rest* kept coming up in your answers over and over again, what can you do to slow down and relax more? If the words *tense* or *tightness* came up a bunch of times, what can you do to unwind? Can you try doing yoga, getting a massage, or simply taking a quiet bath? Take it day by day—it takes time to truly be in tune with your body. Practice honoring yourself this month and it will become second nature to you in no time.

Soothing Spa Solutions

Many women enjoy spa time as part of their self-care routine. You don't have to spend loads of cash or deal with a large amount of products to feel relaxed. The following simple recipes are all you need to create your own at-home spa on a budget, using natural, feel-good ingredients. Essential oils are a great way to help you find calm and recharge during pregnancy. Quality essential oils found in natural food markets can seem expensive, but they last a long time. A few drops are very potent, so be sure to follow directions carefully.

Here are some of my favorite oils that I use with my clients and how they can help you find inner calm and a little relief from outside stress. You can use these oils every day—they are completely safe for you and your baby. Play around with scents you like. Remember, your preferences may change as your senses shift during pregnancy.

- Bergamot: uplifting and antidepressant
- Chamomile: a relaxing, calming sleep aid
- Geranium (after Month Three): uplifting and energizing
- Grapefruit: energizing
- Lavender: relaxing and calming
- Lemon: energizing and purifying
- Neroli: anxiety reducing
- Orange: refreshing and uplifting

- Rosewood: calming, aids with sleep
- Sandalwood: calms and quiets the mind, antidepressant
- Vetiver: reduces anxiety, fights fatigue, antidepressant
- Ylang-ylang: a stress buster

Recharging Bath Meditation

You'll need:

- Essential oils. Try lavender, sweet orange, and peppermint. This pleasant-smelling blend of oils promotes relaxation, lifts the spirits, and helps with morning sickness. Of course, if your nose can't take any of these smells, feel free to test out other scents. Play around with the scents in the following recipes, depending on your mood and what you most need help with (like sleep, focus, or calm).
- 2 cups Epsom salts

In a dry bathtub, add 15 drops of lavender oil, 10 drops of sweet orange oil, and 3 drops of peppermint oil to the Epsom salts. Fill the bathtub with warm water, get in the tub, and begin to breathe deeply.

Concentrate on the lavender smell when breathing in. Feel your body relax, and let go of your tension when you exhale. Next, breathe in the scent of orange, and feel your body let go of any fear or worry. Finally, take in the scent of peppermint and feel it energizing you and releasing any nausea and/or fatigue.

Breathe in this calming aroma and, with every exhale, feel the bath melt away tension, stress, or fatigue that you've been carrying around with you. Imagine this energy coming out of your pores and going into the tub, as if the oils were pulling it out of you like a magnet. When you empty the tub, imagine all the stressful energy flowing from your body as it disappears down the drain with the rest of the bathwater.

Simple Lemon-Sugar Scrub

I already wrote about how amazing lemon is at helping keep morning sickness at a minimum. When it's time to pamper yourself, here's another lemon-based recipe that will keep your skin soft and smelling fresh. This scrub will last you 2 to 3 months if kept in a cool, dark place.

1 cup sugar (any kind)

6 drops lemon essential oil

Juice and peel of 1 lemon

¼ cup coconut oil

1 small mason jar

In a large bowl, combine the sugar, essential oil, and freshly squeezed lemon juice. Mix in the coconut oil. (Add more if you like a wet consistency.) Add the lemon peel. Pour the lemon-sugar mixture into the jar.

Use the scrub in the shower, after washing. Gently rub it on your skin and rinse with warm water.

Soothing Lavender Face Mask

Yogurt is a natural food with many health benefits, both inside the body and out. Yogurt has a smooth consistency and hydrating elements that make it the perfect base for homemade face masks. Honey soothes the skin and kills any bacteria that may be lurking on it.

2 tablespoons plain yogurt (I like Greek yogurt for a thicker consistency)

1 teaspoon honey (organic, if possible)

3 or 4 drops lavender oil

⅓ teaspoon dried lavender flowers

In a small bowl, combine the yogurt, honey, oil, and lavender. Smooth the mixture all over your face and neck. Lie down or sit in a quiet place for 10 minutes, breathing in the soothing lavender smell. Finally, rinse off the mask with warm water and moisturize your skin like you normally would.

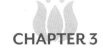

CHAPTER 3

Month Three

EMBRACE YOUR AUTHENTIC SELF

"Be yourself. Everyone else is already taken."

—Oscar Wilde

Not only does pregnancy transform your body for 9 months, but having a baby also opens up an entirely new set of questions about who you are as a person, soon-to-be parent, and role model. This is a great time to explore who you *truly* are, rather than be who people *expect* you to be. Now that you're having a baby, think of it this way: Even though your child comes into this world with her own soul and life path, she's still directly related to you—and how you express yourself affects the way your child will grow and develop.

We are all multidimensional beings. All of us have amazing qualities as well as not-so-wonderful aspects—this is what being human is all about. Many people are afraid to explore these different sides, or to express themselves. When you're okay with your strengths *and* weaknesses, you'll be better able to accept, embrace, and appreciate your child's individuality, too. Practice thinking of yourself as a mirror and reflecting self-love, self-expression, self-acceptance, and acceptance of those around you.

When we are first born, we come into this world whole and pure. As time passes and we journey through life, we tend to pick up projections from our parents, society, and peers about how we should live. We get hurt or allow ourselves to be vulnerable, letting our true selves be seen and perhaps not accepted. So we find coping skills and build a false sense of self or identity. For many of us, it's easier to wear masks that we think will make us more acceptable, attractive, and likable than to be exposed to (and possibly shunned by) the world. The real you *wants* and *needs* to be seen and accepted. Yet, if who you are doesn't fit the "normal" standards of those around you, you can be swayed into thinking that something might be wrong with you.

Here's the thing: If you don't accept and embrace all the parts of yourself, both the good and bad, you might try to re-create in your kids the authentic person you aren't comfortable showing the world, instead of allowing them to be who *they* authentically are. Or you could not accept and possibly pass judgment on your kids for showing a uniqueness that you're not accepting of in yourself. For example, say you always wanted to be an artist. Somewhere during your life, your parents told you that you couldn't make a living as an artist, that in order to "make it" you needed a steady job in this or that field. Or someone criticized your work and squashed your plans for the future. Instead of pursuing your dream, you shut down, putting your artistic dreams to the side while following a completely different path.

Now, here you are, about to become a mom! That artistic part needs to be expressed in some way and integrated into your life. Whether you take art classes or paint in your spare time as a hobby, integrating this forgotten or disowned part of yourself back into your life is extremely important. This is all part of your special "stew" that makes you who you truly are. Everyone is unique and has different ingredients and seasonings in her mix. The more seasonings and ingredients you add to your stew, the more authentic and unique it will be.

As your child grows, these special gifts you hold and unique aspects of yourself are what your child will learn from you. *You* are the perfect mother for your child—your child came here to learn certain things that only you, as his mother, can teach him. If you don't integrate and accept these forgotten parts of yourself, you'll naturally tend to try and re-create them in your children. You may unconsciously push your child to take art lessons or go to museums every weekend when she loves soccer and only wants to kick a ball around. The more you can be in your authentic truth, the better able you'll be to divinely guide and support your children in their own authenticity.

In this chapter, I'll help you find ways to explore your authentic self from the inside out. For now, let's talk about everything that's going on physically.

YOUR CHANGING BODY

Whether it's been an easy transition into your pregnancy or you've been run-down and sick, you're in the homestretch of the first trimester. Here's what you may be experiencing during the third month of your pregnancy, and how your baby is forming.

Fatigue and nausea may play a major role in your daily routine, but a lot of internal changes are setting the stage for your next two trimesters. One concerns circulation. During pregnancy, there's a large increase in blood produced in your veins to support both you and your little one. Don't be surprised if people start telling you that you're glowing—you really are! By the end of your first trimester, your hormones and increased bloodflow make your skin blush and look fuller—that's the secret behind the "pregnancy glow."

Heartburn is also common because of the upward movement of the enlarging uterus, which displaces the stomach and can cause acids to back up into the esophagus. Here are some natural solutions to prevent "the burn."

- Eat smaller, more frequent meals throughout the day and chew your food slowly and thoroughly. This can keep your digestive system from working too hard.

- Drink at least one 8-ounce glass of water or coconut water every hour.

- Eat dinner at least 2 hours before going to bed, and avoid eating late at night.

- Avoid lying down after a meal. Staying upright for at least an hour will better allow you to digest your food.

- Keep your head propped up above your heart while lying down.

- Wear clothes that fit loosely around the waist.

- Eat papaya or take papaya enzymes after each meal. Papaya contains digestive enzymes that soothe the stomach to prevent reflux.

- Eat a few spoonfuls of yogurt after meals. The probiotics in yogurt can help neutralize the acids in your stomach and esophagus.

- Avoid chocolate, tomato-based sauces, citrus fruits, caffeinated drinks, garlic, onions, and greasy and spicy foods. These foods all contain acids that can jump-start acid reflux and heartburn.

- Drink chamomile, peppermint, ginger, or fennel tea. You can even try mixing a few teas together—chamomile mixed with peppermint is a yummy combination.

- Place three fingers on the inside of your wrist (where there is a little dip). Press down hard for a few seconds, then let go. Do this 30 times. These pressure points on your wrist help jump-start digestion.

YOUR GROWING BABY

If you were able to see your baby at this point in an ultrasound, you would first notice that his head is much larger than his body. This is the time when your baby's brain is growing rapidly. Your baby's body will become more proportional very soon, but for now it's going through the natural motions of development.

Because of brain development, brain waves can now be measured. The main construction of the heart is complete. Through its parchment-thin skin, the baby's veins are clearly visible. During this month the ears, the teeth, and the palate are continuing to form.

By the end of Month Three, your baby is around 2 inches long and weighs about half an ounce. He is about the size of a lime.

HEARTBURN BREATHING EXERCISES

Forty to 80 percent of women experience some sort of heartburn and indigestion during pregnancy. These simple breathing exercises can help open up the heart and stomach with your breath, allowing your organs to stretch, then relax. Perform them daily to help with indigestion and heartburn. Repeat each pose 5 times.

- Sit with your legs crossed and place your hands on your ankles. Inhale through your nose, feeling the breath in your stomach as you arch your back and look up. Exhale through your mouth as you look down and round your back.

- Next, inhale through your nose as you arch your back, raising your arms over your head at the same time. Exhale through your mouth as you grab your ankles and round your back.

- Still sitting in a cross-legged position, interlace your hands behind you and move them a few inches behind your lower back. As you inhale through your nose, look up. As you exhale through your mouth, look down and squeeze your shoulder blades together.

- For this next exercise, kneel on a bolster or yoga block. Bring your arms behind your back and grab your elbows. Stick your chest out and inhale through your nose, feeling the breath in your heart and stomach. Exhale through your mouth as your shoulders relax.

🖎 Finally, while sitting in a chair, interlace your fingers behind your head and inhale through your nose, feeling the breath move into your stomach and heart. Exhale through your mouth as you press your elbows back and down.

YOUR EYES DURING PREGNANCY

Hormones are the most common cause of vision changes while you're pregnant. The cornea, the front part of your eye, may swell. Dry eyes and puffy eyelids can make contact lenses uncomfortable, and even women who already wear glasses may notice slight changes in vision. After the baby is born and you're done breast-feeding, most of these changes stop and you can go back to wearing contact lenses comfortably.

Here are some simple ways to help rest your eyes and prevent swelling.

🖎 Take breaks from the computer or from reading.

🖎 Use a humidifier to increase the level of moisture reaching your eyes.

🖎 Stay hydrated.

🖎 Wear sunglasses outside to avoid straining your eyes.

🖎 Use preservative-free artificial tears (eyedrops).

🖎 Avoid overexposure to fans, air conditioning, and heating ducts.

🖎 Blink your eyes more to produce more tears and moisturize your eyes.

🖎 Avoid coffee, which is a diuretic and causes acidity in your body.

🖎 Avoid salt, which can make eyes puffy.

- Soak two chamomile tea bags in hot water. Let them cool and place them over your eyes for 10 minutes. The tea works as an anti-inflammatory for your eyes.
- Place cold cucumber slices over each eye. The cucumber adds moisture to your skin and has a nice cooling effect as well.
- Boil 1 cup of water with 1 teaspoon of fennel seeds. Let cool and add three drops of lavender oil to the mixture. Saturate two cotton balls in the liquid and place them on your eyes for 10 minutes. This will help soothe dry eyes.
- Potatoes have astringent properties that help reduce eye irritation. Peel a potato and then slice it in half. Put the potato in the refrigerator or freezer for a bit to chill it. Cover each eye with a potato half for 10 minutes.

TUNING IN

"Be willing to let go of who you think you should be, in order to become who you are."

—Brené Brown

As wonderful as childhood can be, it comes with its challenges. Maybe you were the unpopular kid, the shy girl, or the one who needed more attention than most. Everyone wants the best for her children, to provide them with a happy home, maybe even a better childhood than her own.

I believe that children come into the world with their own souls, special gifts, and unique paths they'll travel in life. It's up to their parents to help guide them by allowing them to be who they are *meant* to be instead of who their parents *think* they should be. When you really tune in to your child and allow her—no matter how young—to express herself, you'll give her a foundation rooted in love and acceptance. When a child is supported for who she is, she will truly shine and flourish.

So many people try to heal their own childhood wounds through their children. I've seen people try to make their children do and be things they wanted to do or be—but couldn't—when they were young. Sometimes I see people (with the best intentions, of course) wanting to give their children things they never had. Just because you wanted something in life doesn't mean that your child necessarily does. One of the best ways to be aware that you're doing this is to ask yourself: Who am I really doing this for?

When you're okay with truly being yourself, then you'll also be okay with your children and other loved ones being who they truly are as well. People who try to change and control others are usually not very comfortable with themselves. So before trying to mold your child into something you want her to be, stop and take a moment to explore what you might need to change, heal, or accept in yourself first.

"Not everyone thinks the way you think, knows the things you know, believes the things you believe, nor acts the way you would act. Remember this and you will go a long way in getting along with people."

—Arthur Forman

Think about how awful it makes you feel when someone tries to mold you into who they think you should be. Now think of a person who simply loves and supports you for who you are and how that makes you feel. When you feel supported, your energy expands, and when you feel dismissed, your energy contracts. If you find yourself constantly trying to mold your children into who you hope or want them to be, maybe it's best to put that energy into accepting yourself, instead.

I remember years ago working with a couple who had one of the most interesting kids I had ever met. He would talk to me passionately about things I never knew much about—butterflies, artists, science experiments, bugs, and the stars. He was only 5 at the time! His father was a big sports fan and had introduced him to soccer and basketball, but the little boy showed no interest. Instead, he just wanted his parents to take him to the library to get a book on metamorphosis or dinosaurs and dig for bugs and explore nature. His father kept pushing sports, but after watching him suffer and not enjoy them the way he did, he took a really good look at himself and realized he wasn't doing this for his child, but for himself.

When this dad stopped and took a *good* look at who this miraculous being was and accepted that this amazing boy was very different than he was, he saw just how special this little guy was in his own way. Instead of soccer or softball, after-school activities became art classes and guitar lessons, and adventures were visits to the aquarium, nature hikes, or science camp. Needless to say, this little boy is thriving in his own authenticity because his parents have allowed him to just be him.

WEARING HATS

My brother told me about a life coach who asked him to think about all of the different "hats" he wore. I love this concept. He wore the hats of a dad, brother, son, black belt, teacher, coach, husband, and friend. The different hats were just different ways to express his energy. I now do this exercise a lot with my clients. After they give birth and come out of the "baby bubble," I help them slowly express all aspects of themselves using this new way of thinking.

I once worked with a mom who said she felt stuck because she was "only" a mom (which, by the way, is one of the most important and rewarding hats of all but is the one that rarely gets enough credit). I tried the hat exercise with her, and by the end of it she was wearing 45 hats! Her hats included those of a wife and mom, of course, but also a photographer and artist. She made an effort to remember the hats she wore and reclaimed so many parts of herself, including expressing herself through her art.

Becoming a mother is like a metamorphosis—your pregnancy gives you time to grow into the mother you'll develop into even more deeply after your child is born. No one can predict how motherhood will look or feel for you, how things that were once important to you won't be, or how things you never thought you would care about will become your main focus. When you have your baby, you'll also birth this new you—it will be time for you to break free from your pregnancy cocoon and emerge as a butterfly. Each hat you wear is like a different color that makes your butterfly wings more beautiful, special, and unique.

MASKS AND SHIFTING ENERGY

"No man, for any considerable period, can wear one face to himself and another to the multitude, without finally getting bewildered as to which may be the true."

—Nathaniel Hawthorne

Just like hats, people also wear masks at some point or another. Masks help conceal how we're feeling, hiding the truth, a belief we have, or a mood we feel. Masks can be worn for a short time or become a part of your daily life. Masks are an illusion, something you wear to hide the real you.

Perhaps you forgot about or hid a part of yourself over time because you weren't comfortable with it. This can lead to wearing a mask to overcompensate for this disowned part of yourself. For example, I was a shy kid and a bit of a wallflower. To cope and fit in, I adopted a huge personality and became very vivacious to mask the shy little girl that I was never comfortable being. But I knew I needed to allow myself to feel shy at times and be okay with it. I have friends who have shy kids, and sometimes it drives them crazy. I often ask them if they were shy at some point. One hundred percent of the time, they say yes. This goes right back to accepting and making peace with all aspects of one's self in order to accept others. What we don't like in others can often be a reflection of a part of ourselves we don't like or want to accept.

Nobody is perfect. But if you are constantly pretending to be someone else, this false sense of self will attract the wrong people. When you wear a mask all the time and don't put the full expression of yourself out into the world, it can shut down your spirit and leave you feeling depressed. Not everyone will understand or like you, but I promise that when you put the real you out there, you will attract the right people in ways that resonate with you. Only when you accept and express the real you will you be able to find the unique parenting style that is carried from your truth. It may not be the way your sister, friends, or mother did it (or think it should be done). Just like we tell children so they grow up confident and authentic: It's okay to be unique and different!

Years ago, I had a friend who lashed out at me in a very judgmental way. I calmly said to him, "Wow, if you're this hard and judgmental about me, I can only imagine how hard you must be on yourself." Again, we can't accept others if we don't accept ourselves first. If you aren't okay with the stuff you are covering up with a mask, you might not be accepting of others, especially your children, if you happen to see these same qualities in them. Think about it: Are you hiding a side of yourself behind a mask? What parts of yourself are you not letting be seen, and why?

Here's the point of all of this talk about your authentic self: You can only wear the mask for so long before the real you is revealed. It's exhausting to be something you're not. The world needs the special gifts and uniqueness that only you can share. People can get so far away from who they truly are that they have no idea who their authentic self is. When you can accept who you are—the good, the bad, and the ugly—only then can you fully accept others for who they really are. This includes the little one who will become the most important person in the world to you, the one you will teach how to live and love and support in finding and accepting himself—your child.

There's also a tactic I call "shifting energy." This is different from a mask because it's a temporary way to change your feelings or mood when it's appropriate. For example, if I'm in a bad mood or not feeling my best and it's time for my client to have her baby, it's not productive for me to bring this kind of energy into the birth space. My client needs to labor well and feed off of my positive energy. I've learned to shift my energy by checking my baggage at the door. When I do this, I'm able to show up in a more positive, focused, and joyful state. I know that when I'm finished, I can pick up my baggage, unpack it, and continue the process of working through it.

Being mindful of how my energy will affect those around me allows me to shift my moods to meet the needs of others. This trick is especially good to remember as a new mom. Just as my clients feed off my energy, so will your children feed off yours. Of course, having feelings and emotions is a part of being human, and it's important to feel and express. I'm saying this so you can be more mindful of how your energy affects those around you.

During labor, you'll be riding the energy of your partner or anyone else you allow in your sacred birth space. It's important that everyone with you also practice this mindful energy shift. Energy is contagious! The calmer and more positive everyone around you is, the more you'll feel the same. All negativity, projections, and fears should be left outside the birth space.

ACCEPTING YOUR STRENGTHS AND WEAKNESSES

"Be who you were created to be and you will set the world on fire."
—St. Catherine of Siena

One part of embracing your authentic self is to recognize your strengths and weaknesses. People with the best intentions will project their views and ways onto you, during pregnancy and beyond. If you don't have a strong sense of self, you'll be easily swayed and confused, doubting your decisions and wondering if they're what you, your partner, and your child really want and need.

We all have strengths and limits that make us who we are. If you aren't honest about what you can handle and who you truly are, you will get swept up in society's and others' projections about how your life should be. There is no one right way to do anything, but there is a right way for you. When you can find your truth, you will be able to stay true to yourself and do what's right for you and your family. When I work with someone, I take the time to really tune in, see who this person is, and tailor my program to her individual needs. When you're comfortable accepting and embracing all the different parts of yourself, you'll be all right with others being who they are. Ultimately, you'll be more confident and able to find your way and do what feels right as you stand strong in your sense of self.

Here are some questions to ask yourself as you continue your pregnancy journey.

- What are your unique and special qualities?
- What makes you different, unlike anyone else in the world?
- What gives you joy and passion?
- Are you expressing and walking your truth, allowing the real you to be seen and heard?
- Where are you playing it safe or holding yourself back from fully putting yourself out there and living life?

Every woman, pregnancy, birth, and child is unique. In all my years as a doula I have never seen the same birth twice—no two women, no relationship, no two newborns are the same. What might have helped your mother or best friend during pregnancy might not be the right thing for you. I highly suggest taking this time to really get to know yourself and be honest with yourself about who you are and what your truth is. You will have tons of people (with the best intentions) projecting their views and ways onto you. If you don't know who you are and what *feels* right for you, you might get carried away listening to others about becoming a new mother. I never treat my clients the same; instead, I tune in to who they are, help them find their truth, and empower them by supporting them in their authentic way.

BURNING THE MAN

The best example I can give you about authentic self relates to the Burning Man festival, which I visited once, years ago. Burning Man is, in a nutshell, a weeklong gathering of 60,000 people from all walks of life, together in the middle of Nevada's Black Rock Desert. For this one week, Burning Man is its own, self-sufficient "city" on an ancient dried-up lakebed. It's a communal effort to create art and celebrate the earth, life, and people. At the end of the week, a giant "Man" is set on fire, an exciting event for everyone to experience together.

I thought Burning Man was going to be a bunch of crazy people running around on drugs, dancing naked in the desert without inhibitions. Well, there was some of that, but what I connected with was much deeper. What I found was that the creativity and self-expression at Burning Man were infectious and incredibly inspiring. Someone told me what Burning Man was about: The burning of the Man is symbolic of who or what holds us back from our true self-expression. Without inhibitions, people at Burning Man were able to let go and be whoever they wanted to be—because nobody there cared. It's about letting go of the mask, the armor, the shield, the junk (represented by the Man) and letting go of all that we have been repressing, so that who we authentically are can come out and be free.

Another amazing part of Burning Man is the sense of community. There's no money to be exchanged for food, water, or anything you need to survive in the middle of the desert. It's all about helping your neighbor and giving unconditionally. Everyone there is friendly and supportive, no matter the age, interests, politics, skin color, or background. I made some wonderful connections with people as well as had some of the deepest and most honest conversations with total strangers, just because we were all being open and living in our truth. There were no guards up, no armor on, and no inhibitions—just people being real.

Can you imagine if we all lived from this place of true authenticity in our daily lives? Where we would be free to be who and what we really are? So many of us don't even know who we *are* because we are so busy trying to be what others *want* us to be. A lot of people fear that if they really express their true selves they won't be liked or accepted. Others have so much stress and negativity in their lives that they don't know that there's an inner light that's waiting to shine big and bright. Still other people are afraid to let go of control. And many are so caught up in fear that they don't know how to get out of their heads and feel and act from their hearts.

I had an amazing opportunity to work with some of the shamans at Burning Man. My companion experienced a huge awakening during a healing session, expressing happiness, positivity, and a lightness through his whole body. I love what the shamans said to him: "Welcome home! This is you. What you are feeling is your self. This is what's under the crap, the junk, the stress, fear, and the persona you've taken on to be accepted by others. What you will find here is your true self."

"Your playing small doesn't serve the world."

—Marianne Williamson

MEDITATION: CREATING A PICTURE OF YOUR AUTHENTIC SELF

You will need a mirror, magazines, a large piece of paper, scissors, and glue.

I know that not everyone is comfortable writing in a journal all the time. Some people are more visual and tactile. For this exercise, I want to feed that visual part of your authentic self. Get into a comfortable, cross-legged position in front of a mirror. Look at yourself—begin to really look into your own eyes. Hold your gaze for a few minutes. Let your thoughts come and go, and acknowledge them without being attached to them. Instead, label them as thinking and bring your attention back to yourself, looking deep into your eyes, to the depth of your soul. Without overthinking, go with whatever pops into your mind, even if it doesn't make sense. Try and take your mind out of the process—be playful and free. Your inner guidance/spirit will take over and will create an image of your happiest being from a place of truth, not your ego or mind.

From here, get your magazines and start to cut out words and pictures representing who is waiting and wanting to come out and be expressed—your authentic self. Be aware of what you're drawn to.

JOURNAL WORK: WHO AM I?

This month, I challenge you to work on "burning the Man" and allowing your truth of who you authentically are to be expressed fully. When you can embrace, accept, honor, and express your truth, others will, too. When you are free and it feels right, you'll know you have found yourself. There will be a sense of joy and peace, and you'll know you are home.

Here are some questions to ask yourself. They may be tough to answer, or you may find you have more than enough to say about the topic. Be honest with yourself and don't hold back. Write down your answers in your journal, or feel free to meditate on your answers in a quiet place in your home.

- Is this person I am putting out there into the world really me?
- If not, why am I not allowing myself to be seen?
- What am I repressing?
- What am I afraid of?
- What thoughts, fears, or beliefs are coming up for me?
- What is holding me back? What shields, masks, armor, and junk (the "Man") are getting in the way of me being my true self?
- Am I ready to let them go and be free?
- What needs to be expressed?
- What needs to burn?

After doing this exercise, either write down or draw on a piece of paper what's preventing you from being yourself—the block, mask, or whatever is holding you back from being free to be the real you. What does this block look and feel like? Are there words or colors associated with what's holding you back? When you're ready, make an intention to let this go so you can be free. Then, burn the paper carefully and in a safe space, such as a sink or fireplace. This is a gesture that you're releasing to the world all that needs to be let go of and freed.

If you see someone cooking and you feel the pull to cook more, then cut out that picture. If a photo of a child or big family appeals to you, cut it out as well. If your heart says you want to be a world traveler someday, find photos of exotic locations or other places that jump out at you and are calling you to visit. Glue them onto the paper any way you want. Afterward, journal about what it feels like to have these interests and goals, and write out ways you can integrate them into your life. Take those next steps and take action!

PREVENTING STRETCH MARKS

Stretch marks are very common during pregnancy. They're the result of rapid weight gain mixed with pregnancy hormones such as progesterone. There's no telling if you'll get them; some women do and others don't.

A few factors determine whether or not someone will develop stretch marks during pregnancy. A lot depends on hereditary factors, so chances are that if your mother had them, most likely you will, too. Darker-skinned women are also more prone to visible stretch marks than lighter-skinned women. Your skin's elasticity has something to do with it, as well as nutrition and diet. An unhealthy diet (high in processed foods) has been linked to contributing to the appearance of stretch marks.

To prevent stretch marks, I suggest my clients start eating a healthy diet full of whole foods as early as possible, as discussed in Chapter 1. You should also make sure to stay well hydrated by drinking plenty of water. I'm a huge fan of coconut water. I also recommend foods rich in good fatty acids. These include fish oil, olive oil, coconut oil, chia seeds, almonds and nut butters, lentils, split peas, wheat germ, salmon, cod, avocados, kale, spinach, collard greens, and winter squash.

There's no miracle cure for stretch marks, but keeping your belly moisturized will allow the skin to stay more elastic and soft. I've created a "belly butter" in my kitchen and recommend it for all of my clients. Made with all-natural oils, the belly butter is easy to make and keep in your bathroom or by your nightstand. Use the belly butter on your breasts, hips, and tummy. As an added bonus, this is a great after-bath, all-over body moisturizer for the whole family, even people with sensitive skin. Kids will go crazy for it since it smells like chocolate—if you can be convinced to share!

Breggy's All-Natural Belly Butter

2 glass jars organic coconut oil

1 cup raw organic cocoa butter

½ cup raw organic shea butter

1 bottle (0.5 ounce) liquid vitamin E oil

Melt the coconut oil by placing the glass jars in hot water in a large pan on the stove until the oil liquefies.

Pour the liquid coconut oil into another pot. Add the cocoa butter, shea butter, and vitamin E and stir until melted together. Pour the mixture back into the coconut oil jars. You will have some extra that you can put into an additional glass jar.

The mixture will harden when it cools. Keep one jar in a cool space (under your sink, for example) and use it regularly. I always store the remaining jars in the refrigerator so the belly butter doesn't spoil. There are no preservatives, but this will keep for a few months.

Here's a great meditation you can try while using this belly butter on your skin. With our lives being so busy, sometimes it's hard to make time to connect with your baby. Take a few moments while you're getting ready for your day or before bed to make this conscious connection between your body and your baby.

◈ Place some belly butter in your hands. Rub your hands together and place them on your belly. Breathe in, deep into your belly, and take a moment to acknowledge your pregnancy and body and how amazing it is that you are creating the miracle of life inside.

- Next, begin to rub the butter all around your belly. Feel the gratitude you have for this baby you're carrying and all your joy and excitement. Think about how your baby is growing and visualize him changing and moving around. As your pregnancy progresses and you read more about all of the incredible changes your baby is going through, feel gratitude for the process for both you and your soon-to-be child.

- Feel free to also rub the belly butter on your breasts and hips! Again, feel gratitude and awe for the milk you're able to make and for your hips expanding to birth your baby with ease.

KEGELS FOR PREGNANCY AND BEYOND

Kegels are a simple exercise to strengthen your pelvic floor muscles, providing benefits throughout pregnancy and beyond. If you're not already doing Kegel exercises, start now. The squeezing motion of Kegels improves circulation to both your vaginal and rectal areas. Here's what they can do for you.

- Prevent or treat urinary incontinence (peeing a little when you sneeze or cough), which affects up to 70 percent of women during and after pregnancy

- Reduce the risk of anal incontinence

- Help with pelvic pain as your pregnancy progresses

- Keep hemorrhoids away

- Speed up healing after an episiotomy or tear during childbirth

- Improve the muscle tone of your vagina (meaning sex will feel better)

You can do Kegels anywhere—in the shower, at work, while cooking or waiting in line for something—and no one will know! For Kegels to be effective, you need to do a lot of them every day, around 30 to 40 squeezes. One trick I tell my clients is to do Kegels every time they're sitting at a red light. If you live in a high-traffic area like I do, you'll be done with your daily Kegels in no time.

Here's how to get your Kegels done the right way.

- **Locate your pelvic muscles.** Pretend you're tightening your vagina around a tampon or stop peeing midstream. Both actions involve the pelvic muscles.

- **Practice in various positions.** Lying on your back might work until you get the feel of contracting the pelvic floor muscles. Afterward, you can do your Kegels sitting and standing, too.

- **Practice Kegel "contractions."** You'll want to master both short contractions and releases and longer ones, increasing the strength of the contraction and holding it at a maximum for up to 10 seconds. Long contractions will take more practice. Relax the pelvic muscles between repetitions, and hold the relaxation phase for the same amount of time as the contraction. Start by holding each contraction for 3 to 5 seconds, resting the same number of seconds in between. Build up to 10-second contractions, with 10 seconds of rest between contractions.

- **Keep your other muscles relaxed.** When doing pelvic floor exercises, don't contract your abdominal, leg, or buttock muscles or lift your pelvis. It's easier to keep these other muscles relaxed when standing or lying on your side, with no pressure on other parts of your body.

GETTING YOUR GROOVE ON

Some women *love* sex while they're pregnant and can't get enough of it, while others can't stand the thought of it. As long as you're having a healthy pregnancy, you can have sex as often as you'd like. Sex is an amazing way for you and your partner to bond and connect. Here are a few great reasons to have sex during pregnancy.

- During pregnancy, the increase of bloodflow causes engorgement of the genitals, which can increase the intensity of an orgasm. There's also an increase in vaginal discharges, which makes for an awesome lubricant, heightening sensations during sex.

- Sexual activity increases intimacy with your partner, as well as keeps you in tune with your own body. It also gives your partner a chance to explore your body in an intimate setting.

- Having an orgasm releases the hormone oxytocin, which helps boost your mood, lowers blood pressure, reduces pain, and boosts your immune system.

- Releasing energy during sex helps you relax and sleep better.

If you're just not into sex and feel sick, emotional, and tired, there's nothing like a great snuggle session. Here are some benefits of hugging.

- Hugging increases oxytocin and serotonin levels, which elevates your mood, increases happiness, and eases depression. It also relaxes your muscles and helps relieve tension and pain in your body.

- Being close to your partner reduces stress.

- Hugging promotes a sense of security with your partner.

- Recent medical research at the University of North Carolina found that both blood pressure and levels of cortisol, the hormone we produce when under stress, were significantly lowered (particularly in women) when subjects hugged their partners for at least 20 seconds.

BLOOD BUILDERS

Anemia during pregnancy is a result of a deficiency of iron in the blood. Every red blood cell in your body uses iron to help carry hemoglobin—the oxygen-carrying component of blood—to you and your baby. Your body needs much more iron than normal when you're pregnant (and breastfeeding, later on). Around 20 percent of women experience anemia during pregnancy, but many women don't feel any symptoms. A simple blood test performed by your doctor can tell you if you're anemic.

Some symptoms of anemia are:

- Loss of appetite
- Fatigue and/or lethargy
- Irritability
- Breathlessness
- Headaches or dizziness
- Depression
- Sore tongue
- Cracks in the corners of your mouth
- Cold hands or feet
- Pale skin/pallor
- Brittle nails

Iron is not produced naturally by the body and needs to be absorbed into the system through food and supplements. Since your body is naturally producing more blood as your pregnancy goes on, you'll want it to be as nutrient-rich for your baby as possible. Eating iron-rich foods is the most effective way to get iron into your system safely and naturally, but there are other ways to sneak iron into your body. Here are some great foods and tips to get iron into your system, and better yet, your baby-to-be.

- Avoid coffee, eggs, milk, and bran. These foods can inhibit the absorption of iron. It's okay to eat them well before or after taking a supplement, but eating them at the same time will diminish iron absorption.

- Lower stomach acid levels, caused by taking antacids, can also lower iron absorption. Ask your doctor about taking antacids for heartburn or acid reflux.

- I like Floradix liquid iron supplement. It's absorbed faster than a supplement in pill form. Take Floradix with orange juice or vitamin C.

- Foods that are high in iron can build the blood and correct anemia. These include liver, ground beef, lamb, whole wheat bread, beans, lentils, peas, potatoes, pomegranates, apricots, bee pollen, blackberries, cherries, eggs, figs, dark green leafy vegetables, prunes, raisins, red meat, and seaweeds.

- Vitamin C improves the absorption of iron. You'll want to get the vitamin naturally by eating vitamin C–rich foods such as grapefruit, oranges or orange juice, vegetable or tomato juice, strawberries, blackberries, raspberries, mangos, cantaloupe, papayas, tomatoes, red or green peppers, cabbage, broccoli, cauliflower, and leafy greens.

- Try this morning anemia-fighting drink: Mix lemon juice or apple cider vinegar with a little honey in the morning. You can also start your day by having a glass of warm water with honey and lemon. Honey helps build hemoglobin levels in the body and also provides energy and strength.

- Bananas and honey have a rich supply of iron. Mash a banana and eat it with a bit of honey one or two times a day. I also put this on brown rice cakes for a great afternoon snack.

- Try reflexology, which uses pressure points on your feet to stimulate organs. For anemia, you'll want to find the pressure point for the spleen. The spleen recycles iron and plays an important role in the manufacturing of hemoglobin. I highly recommend going to a professional reflexologist to try this method.

- Almonds are a great source of iron. Soak a few almonds in water every night, peel off the skin in the morning, and eat the almonds raw. Doing this regularly for 3 months could work wonders.

- Beets are also known to be very helpful in curing anemia. Raw beets and beet juice contain a lot of minerals and nutrients. The high iron content in a beetroot helps in the formation of red blood cells.

- Soak 2 to 15 raisins overnight in water. Eat them with a bit of honey the next morning, with breakfast. Do this every day for a month. Eating raisins and honey is a natural way to get iron. You can also eat three or four figs every day.

- Use cast-iron pans for cooking. Foods cooked in cast iron can absorb the iron from the pans.

- For vegetarians, a great iron tonic is 1 tablespoon brewer's yeast, 1 tablespoon wheat germ, 1 tablespoon blackstrap molasses,

1 tablespoon canola oil, and 4 ounces orange juice. Drink this one to three times daily.

- Blackstrap molasses is a home remedy frequently recommended for anemia. Take 1 tablespoon twice a day. Or mix together 2 teaspoons of apple cider vinegar and 2 teaspoons of blackstrap molasses, add the mixture to water or tea, and drink.

- Drink strong teas throughout the day, alternating between nettle and red raspberry leaf. To make your own tea, steep an ounce of freeze-dried or fresh nettle leaf in a quart of boiled water for at least 4 hours and drink ½ to 1 cup several times daily.

- Seaweed (kelp and/or dulse) is another good source of iron; you can put kelp powder in soup or take six kelp tablets daily.

- Bottled chlorophyll is another alternative. Take 1 to 3 table-spoons per day, depending on your individual requirements.

EATING NATURALLY FOR ENERGY

The third month can still be a challenging time, especially if you're battling fatigue. If your nausea hasn't abated, you may still be unable to get a lot of foods down. Thankfully, there are plenty of foods to naturally boost your energy. When it comes to feeding your baby this month, keep up with a balanced diet rich in everything. I teamed up with Beaming in LA to create the ultimate pregnancy smoothie. With all the food aversions and crazy cravings during pregnancy, it can be challenging to get something healthy into your body. Lisa (the owner of Beaming) and I came up with the perfect solution! This smoothie is not only delicious, it's jam-packed with superfoods that help both mama and baby. If you're having a tough time eating, try drinking this once a day, and you'll know you're getting a great nutritional boost. You can find the Beaming protein powder and other smoothie kits at livebeaming.com.

The Beaming & Lori Bregman's "Knocked Up" Smoothie

8 ounces almond milk

2 ounces coconut water

1 date

1 tablespoon almond butter

½ cup spinach

¼ avocado

1 tablespoon goji berries

2 tablespoons protein powder (I recommend the Beaming Organic Raw Plant-Based Superfood Protein Blend)

1 teaspoon Beaming Superfood Smoothie Blend (available at livebeaming.com)

1 teaspoon chia powder

½ teaspoon E3Live Original liquid supplement (available at e3live.com), optional

¼ cup frozen banana

½ cup frozen strawberries

1 cup ice

1 tablespoon hemp seeds

Place the almond milk, coconut water, date, almond butter, spinach, avocado, goji berries, protein powder, greens, chia powder, liquid supplement (if using), banana, strawberries, and ice in a blender, and blend on high speed until fully combined. Top with the hemp seeds for extra protein.

You can check your iron levels at home without any special equipment. Pay close attention to how you feel. If you often feel weak, light-headed, and extremely short of breath, these may be warning signs. To check your eyes, look in a mirror and pull down your lower eyelid. The inside of your eyelid should be red or dark pink. A light pink or pale color indicates an iron deficiency.

Here's why the ingredients in this smoothie are good for you.

- According to a study in the *Journal of Obstetrics and Gynecology,* women who ate **dates** daily for their entire pregnancy were more dilated when labor began, less likely to need medication to get labor going, and experienced on average 7 fewer hours of labor than non–date eaters. The study found a compound in the dates that imitates oxytocin (which helps with labor). Dates are also high in iron, a natural energy booster, and great for relieving constipation.

- **Bananas** help your nerves and muscles function properly and are rich in iron and high in fiber, which helps battle constipation and diarrhea. According to a study from Rush University in Chicago, the B vitamins in bananas also help fight depression and improve mood. In addition, bananas are a natural source of energy, help prevent heartburn, and help the body maintain a proper balance of electrolytes.

- **Spinach** helps prevent birth defects thanks to its high folate content. Spinach also protects against cell mutation and cleanses the body of toxins, and it has a laxative effect and is great for easing constipation.

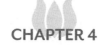

CHAPTER 4

Month Four

DESTRESS AND DECOMPRESS

"If you get the inside right, the outside will fall into place."

—Eckhart Tolle

In my practice as a pregnancy coach and a doula, I believe the calmer a woman feels during her pregnancy, the calmer and more at peace her baby within will be. The fourth month of pregnancy is a time when subtle yet important changes occur, including your belly expanding, possibly feeling the first movement from your baby, and more. Learning how to fully relax and develop an inner peace and calm about yourself and your pregnancy will help immensely in the months and years ahead.

YOUR CHANGING BODY

Welcome to the second trimester! Now may be the time you start telling people about your pregnancy. You may also be feeling a lot better physically than just a few weeks ago. The second trimester is often what people call the "golden" period of pregnancy—many women feel much better overall, are not as uncomfortable, and enjoy the excitement of sharing the news of a new baby on the way. Enjoy this time, and take advantage of feeling better.

Some women (not all) are noticeably pregnant now, as their waistline disappears and muscles and ligaments begin to relax and help support a new body shape. Your appetite may increase as you begin to feel better. Continue to eat healthfully, and watch your portion sizes to ensure optimal nutrition for you and your growing baby.

You may start to feel a slight sensation in your lower abdomen (called quickening). This feels like bubbles or fluttering, and it's an amazing way to start to connect with your baby. And get ready—quickening is very exciting, but the real fun is when those kicks and elbows start coming like lightning. You may not have had to change to maternity pants just yet, but by Month Four, you'll probably want to switch to looser clothing. You also may be ready for a maternity bra, which provides much better support.

At this stage, you may notice changes in skin pigmentation on your face, breasts, and arms, and your nipples and areolas may darken. These are all normal parts of pregnancy and will disappear either before you give birth or soon after. These changes can take many forms, including:

- A dark line running from your navel to your pubic area
- Darkening of existing moles or freckles, or the appearance of new moles
- Blotchy patches on your legs, caused by decreased circulation and an increase in estrogen

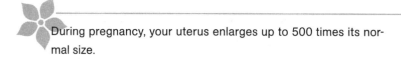

During pregnancy, your uterus enlarges up to 500 times its normal size.

The second trimester is also about expansion, and not just of your growing belly. Your breasts will continue to grow, due to the milk-producing glands prepping for a newborn. You may still experience breast tenderness or soreness, or your breasts may just seem larger now. Don't be surprised if your blood pressure is lower than usual starting now—it's totally normal, especially through the first 6 months of pregnancy. You may be tested for anemia, to see if you're getting enough iron to help your body make enough red blood cells. (As discussed in Chapter 3, untreated anemia can increase your risk of preterm delivery and your baby's risk of low birth weight.)

Hormones are working their way into every system of your body. Progesterone is increasing your lung capacity, and you'll be inhaling and exhaling around 40 percent more air than usual. The oxygen is continuing to support all that blood you're pumping around your body and to baby.

At this point, your uterus is also expanding rapidly, filling with amniotic fluid to make room for your growing baby. While your uterus grows, your belly will also start to expand. This will change your center of gravity, and you may notice yourself losing your balance and shifting your posture more often. Finally, your growing uterus is putting pressure on your other organs, as well as your veins. Don't worry if you feel more aches and pains in your lower belly and pelvic region—this is all normal and expected.

While you may have been dealing with a sensitive nose or morning sickness, during the fourth month you can start to experience "round ligament pain" in your belly, groin, or pelvic area. These aches and pains are the result of your uterus beginning to stretch your ligaments. It can feel like a dull jabbing or ache and is most commonly felt on the right side of the body. The pain can be uncomfortable, but it's completely normal. Here are some ways you can relieve round ligament pain.

- Sit in lukewarm baths with Epsom salts.

- Avoid sudden movements. If you have to sneeze, laugh, or cough, hugging the affected area of the body can help.

- To relieve some of the pressure on your pelvic area, place your hands under your belly and gently lift upward.

- Lie on your left side with pillows under your belly and between your knees.

- Place a few drops of lavender oil on a heating pad or warm compress and apply it to your lower belly, groin, or the right side of your abdomen.

- Avoid staying in the same position for too long.

- Ask your caregiver about taking over-the-counter pain relievers.

- Wear a pregnancy belt or support for your belly, again, to keep pressure off of your pelvic area.

- Speak with a chiropractor about an adjustment.

It's a very busy month for your body, and it's equally exciting for your baby. Let's take a peek inside at the changes creating your up-and-coming newborn.

YOUR GROWING BABY

A lot of crucial mechanisms are in the final stages of development within your baby during Month Four. Your baby's various internal systems will be almost fully formed at this point, and they'll also function together for the first time. By the end of the fourth month, your baby is 5 to 6 inches long and weighs about 4 ounces (think avocado). Her bones become stronger, allowing her to make movements that you'll soon feel as tiny kicks from your belly. This is also the month when your baby's gender is defined—it's up to you to decide whether to find out or keep it a secret.

In fact, your baby is actually starting to look like—a baby! The beauty of all of this rapid growth is that, while tiny and new, these systems are already beginning to work in sync. Fingers and toes are now well defined, and because muscles and skin are forming, your baby can perform new feats such as making a fist, putting her thumb in her mouth, and making facial expressions. The skeletal system is also beginning to hook up with the nervous system, allowing for better movement coordination.

SHORT- AND LONG-TERM EFFECTS OF STRESS AND ANXIETY

"It's not the load that breaks you down, it's the way you carry it."

—Lena Horne

Many studies have been done to see if stress hormones in a mother's body reach the baby in utero. One study, published in the journal *Current Directions in Psychological Science*, explains that when a pregnant woman is chronically stressed or experiences extreme stress, the baby may be exposed to unhealthy levels of stress hormones, which can impact brain development. Chronic or extreme maternal stress may also cause changes in the blood-flow to the baby, making it difficult for oxygen and other important nutrients to reach the baby's developing organs. Chronically

During birth, a baby will get its first major dose of bacteria as it passes through the birth canal. The baby ingests the mother's vaginal microbes, which will begin to grow and thrive in the newborn's gut. Research presented at an annual Society for Neuroscience meeting explained how a study with mice found that the more stressed-out mice produced a larger variety of bacteria and less of the "good" bacteria. Their babies received less of the essential bacteria at a crucial point—at birth.

or severely stressed mothers may also feel overwhelmed and fatigued, which can impact their diet, sleep habits, and consistency of prenatal care.

In addition, maternal stress and anxiety during pregnancy can have both immediate and long-term effects on newborns. High levels of stress can cause you to experience high blood pressure, which increases your chance of having preterm labor or a low-birth-weight infant. Maternal stress can even lead to an increased risk of miscarriage, according to a study published in the *Proceedings of the National Academy of Science* online journal.

Here are some ways serious stress can affect your baby.

- Smaller birth weight and length
- Temperament problems and colic
- Problems with attention, attention regulation, and emotional reactivity
- Lower scores on measures of mental development

I once flew out of town to work with a woman who was going through an extremely stressful time. When I got there, she

A study from the journal *PLOS ONE* suggests that eating at least some fish during pregnancy may lower your risk of anxiety. Around 9,500 pregnant women were surveyed about their diets during pregnancy. Women who never or rarely ate fish such as tuna and salmon were more likely to have anxiety in their third trimester of pregnancy, compared with women who ate fish at least once a week. This outcome was attributed to the omega-3 fatty acids in fish.

According to the Mayo Clinic, seafood that is low in mercury and high in omega-3s includes salmon, anchovies, herring, sardines, trout, and mackerel. The United States Food and Drug Administration (FDA) recommends that pregnant women eat up to 12 ounces of fish per week (about two meals' worth).

wanted to go to the doctor to get an ultrasound to make sure that everything was okay with the baby. At the time, she was about 11 weeks pregnant. I couldn't believe what I saw on the ultrasound. It looked as though her little baby was doing backflips and jumping jacks in the womb. The energy of this little baby matched his mother's.

Don't get me wrong—just because your baby is active doesn't mean he is stressed. Babies move all the time, some more than others. But this was different; I could feel this baby's stress after seeing him on the screen. Considering what was going on in his mom's life, I wasn't surprised at what we saw on the ultrasound. During the week I spent with her, we did hours of life coaching, yoga, breathwork and meditation, massage, healthy eating, and sleeping. After that 1 week, she wanted to check with the doctor again to make sure her baby was okay. This time the baby was just calmly floating, only once in a while peacefully moving. Even the doctor commented that it looked like a different baby was in there.

Think about how stress affects your body. When you're worried about something—your job, a relationship, finances, etc.—how does your body respond? Does your heart race? Does your stomach or throat tighten? Do you have trouble sleeping? Stress affects your body, mind, and behavior in many ways, some of which you may not even realize. How often do you experience the following?

Physical stress symptoms:

- Headache
- Upset stomach
- Muscle aches
- Fatigue/problems sleeping
- Loss of sex drive

Stress symptoms that affect mood:

- Irritability
- Depression
- Anxiety
- Restlessness
- Lack of focus

Stressful behaviors:

- Overeating
  (or undereating)
- Social withdrawal
- Emotional outbursts
  toward friends or
  loved ones

Well, your baby is as much a part of you as your internal organs. Just as your body and overall well-being are affected by stress, your baby is, too. Stress tightens your body, constricting bloodflow to body parts and organs and, while you're pregnant, to your baby as well. When tension sets in, the energy flow of your body gets stuck and stagnates.

Let's be real about this: Nobody is 100 percent stress-free. Having a stressful moment, day, week, or even few weeks won't have a long-term effect on your child. Being in a constant state of stress, however, could.

STRESS RELIEF

"We don't realize that, somewhere within us all, there does exist a supreme self who is eternally at peace."

—Elizabeth Gilbert

There are ways to lessen the effects of stress. Here are some ways that I suggest to help my clients navigate and release stress during pregnancy.

- Get help controlling stressful situations. Seek support from someone you trust and can count on. This could be your partner, parents, a therapist or life coach, a support group, or friends. Your go-to person should be someone with whom you feel safe sharing your feelings or someone who can support and guide you in a healthy way.
- Get consistent prenatal care from your caregiver. Regular checkups with your health-care professional will help you understand what's going on with your body, and she should be able to answer any questions about your pregnancy that are causing anxiety.

- Get regular exercise. Walk, swim—anything that keeps your body moving regularly. See Chapter 1 for the benefits of exercising during pregnancy.

- Get adequate rest. Try to get a good 8 hours of sleep each night, more if possible. If your body and being feel tired, honor where you are and rest. By resting, you're not "doing nothing"—you're recharging your batteries. People often say they have so much to do that it's impossible to rest. I say that if you can unplug for a bit, you will be a lot more energized, clearheaded, and focused, and thus better able to actually finish what you need to do.

- Follow healthy eating habits. Avoid alcohol, tobacco, and certain prescription medications. Check with your caregiver regarding which prescription medications (as well as over-the-counter meds) are safe to take and which to avoid.

CONSTIPATION CONTROL

With all the hormonal changes going on in your system, you may be experiencing constipation. Constipation is also the result of not getting enough fiber and water in your diet. Being regular while you're pregnant is important. It keeps your system moving and eliminates toxins that build up in your body. The symptoms of constipation include painful bloating, gas, and a general feeling of heaviness.

My number one recommendation is to drink *lots* of fluids. You need to drink at least half a gallon of water, coconut water, fresh juices, or tea per day. As I've said throughout the book, water and hydration in general are essential for staying healthy during pregnancy. In Chapter 1, I give a lot of suggestions for making water more exciting, so check back and try some ways to spice up your water.

Here are more ways to avoid constipation.

- Take alfalfa tablets or drink alfalfa tea. Alfalfa can help with a lot of pregnancy symptoms, like morning sickness, heartburn,

(continued on page 100)

JOURNAL WORK: IDENTIFYING YOUR STRESS

"The greatest weapon against stress is our ability to choose one thought over another."

—**William James**

There are so many different kinds and levels of stress, from emotional, physical, and mental to short-term, long-term, or chronic stress. Everyone reacts to and handles stress differently. Life isn't always easy! How we handle stressful situations can affect our health and well-being, as well as the health of those we live and interact with. I've found many ways to help manage stress.

I love journaling, especially when I'm stressed or going through a hard time. Journaling allows all of my emotions to flow out of my body, and I get to process them on paper in front of me. When you keep your feelings and thoughts inside, they seem bigger and are harder to process and make sense of. Writing about them helps to release the stressful energy and emotions that are stuck in your body and mind and gets them on paper

Before you can resolve your stress by writing about it, you first have to figure out what's causing you to feel stressed. Write out what you're feeling—don't hold back, just let it rip! Even if you feel overwhelmed by all that you need to get done, putting it on paper is a great beginning. You can make a to-do list or write one long sentence; it doesn't need to be grammatically correct or a masterpiece of literature. However you can get your thoughts on paper, get them out there. Remember, this is a personal purging exercise for your eyes only. You can write this on the computer as if you're writing an e-mail and then delete it after you get it all out. If you're upset with someone, write an e-mail to him without sending it. Again, this is just to help you unleash and process your feelings and emotions, instead of potentially lashing out at or putting your issues on others.

How is your ongoing stress making you feel? When I get stressed my jaw and stomach tighten and hurt, I don't eat, and I get an overall feeling of anxiety. Make a list of any physical ailments or symptoms you experience due to stress. They can include tightness in the stomach, a short temper, headaches, nausea, insomnia, and more. I often find that people are so disconnected from their emotions that just a simple check-in to ask themselves what emotions they're feeling right now—or doing the body scan from Chapter 2 (see page 57)—is enough to identify what isn't working.

Get to the root of your emotion: After doing the body scan from Chapter 2, notice where you are physically holding your tension. Begin to breathe and meditate on the spot where your tension lives, visualizing it on or in your body. The first time I tried this exercise, I realized I was holding tension in my throat and I envisioned hands around my neck. Next, see if you can remove or undo the tension block through visualization. When I went deeper into my vision, I removed the hands from my neck. I saw energy coming out of me. I went even deeper into my feelings and I found anger and sadness. An overwhelming feeling came over me, and I wanted to cry and scream. From there, I journaled how I felt. After my "scream" on paper, my whole throat relaxed and softened.

Another example: When working on managing stress with one of my clients, she saw a hard ball in her hip, which was causing her pain. To rid herself of the hard ball (loosen her tension and pain), she visually peeled the ball off her hip and saw a gaping hole. She went deeper into her meditation and felt loneliness and fear after seeing the hole. I had her write from that place of loneliness and fear, to get it all out of her body. She ended up having a good cry as she wrote, and then her hip let go of its pain.

constipation, and anemia. It raises the vitamin K levels of pregnant women (reducing the quantity and duration of postpartum bleeding). Start slowly when taking alfalfa. Try taking one tablet the first day, then two the second day, and so on, until you're taking two tablets after each meal and two before bed. Check with your caregiver before taking alfalfa, as women on blood thinners may not be able to use it.

- Drink lemon and hot water first thing in the morning to wake up your digestive system. Squeeze half a lemon into 8 to 10 ounces of hot water.

- Avoid refined carbohydrates, cheese, and fried or fatty foods. These are foods that clog you up and prevent your bowels from moving.

- Eat more fruits and vegetables, greens, nuts, seeds, dried fruit, yogurt, fiber-rich foods, bran, oats, and whole grains. These are foods that pass through your system more easily.

- Sprinkle flaxseeds or chia seeds on your breakfast cereal or grains.

- Eat a tablespoon of coconut oil before bed to help soften the next morning's stools.

- Soak raisins in water overnight and add them to your cereal.

- Soak a few figs in a glass of half milk/half water for an hour or more. Bring the mixture to a boil for a few minutes. Then drink the warm milk/water mixture before bed. This is a way to bring the syrup out of figs, which are a natural laxative. You can also buy fig syrups, but most have added senna, which is a laxative you want to avoid while pregnant.

- Take an acidophilus supplement.

- Replenish your electrolytes with products such as Ultima Replenisher, a naturally sweetened electrolyte powder you can add to your water.

- Exercise daily.

- Take homeopathic nux vomica 6x three times a day.

- Firmly massage your belly with my belly butter (see page 80). Start at the bottom of your belly and move in a clockwise direction. Continue the massage for 5 to 10 minutes.

- Have your partner massage your lower back firmly with lavender oil, or get a relaxing professional massage.

- Take a bath with an added teaspoon of grapeseed oil and three or four drops of essential oil such as bergamot, sweet orange, or lemon. Relax in the bath and massage your belly in the water to help move your bowels.

- Make sure you have enough time to go to the bathroom and sit on the toilet every day.

- Try squatting on the toilet or elevating your feet. Use a low stool to put your feet up to relieve the pressure on your legs.

- Go when you have the urge—don't hold it in and wait. If your body is telling you to go, *go*.

EAT HAPPY

Did you know that there are many "mood-boosting" foods? Eat these mood-elevating foods and you'll feel better, naturally! A banana, one piece of dark chocolate, tea with honey, even oatmeal are all great mood boosters and help calm your nerves.

Lentils are also a fantastic kitchen staple. They're a complex carbohydrate, so like bananas they have the added benefit of helping to increase the brain's production of the feel-good neurotransmitter serotonin. This results in a calmer, happier state of mind with less anxiety.

Finally, Brazil nuts are the number one source of the mineral selenium, which helps maintain your mood and prevent depression. Scientists aren't sure why, but it seems that selenium is essential for maintaining a happy mood. Just six Brazil nuts give you your recommended daily intake.

- Calcium and magnesium are great minerals to help with constipation, both naturally and slowly. Try drinking Natural Calm powdered drink before bed for best results.

- Taking iron can cause constipation. If you need an iron supplement to help with anemia, try to find an herbal iron source such as Floradix liquid iron supplement, which contains a balance of iron and herbs.

My Favorite Go-To Constipation Cocktail

Here's my favorite easy-to-make-at-home constipation cocktail to help relieve constipation. It's tasty and works naturally. You won't shock your system with this drink.

4 pitted, stewed prunes (soaked in water or apple juice overnight)

2 cups (or more, depending on desired thickness) apple juice

1 tablespoon psyllium husk or bran (If you use bran, soak it in apple juice or water until it's soft before blending.)

1 tablespoon chlorophyll

1 teaspoon flaxseeds

In a blender, combine the prunes, apple juice, psyllium husk, chlorophyll, and flaxseeds. Blend until smooth, adding more apple juice as needed to achieve the desired thickness.

Drink 8 to 12 ounces of water right away after drinking this constipation cocktail, to help your system digest it. You can also heat up the cocktail, like warm cider, or add less juice and make it more of a mush that you eat with a spoon.

YOGA FOR CONSTIPATION

Constipation is most often attributed to certain foods, insufficient water intake, and pregnancy hormones building up in your body. Did you know that constipation can also be a result of stress and an inability to let go? If you did the journal work from earlier in the chapter, you may have identified what factors are stressing you out. For this next exercise, think about what you may be holding on to or unable to let go of in your life. This will be helpful during birth, as you *must* be able to let go to birth your baby.

Breathwork for Constipation Relief

Try this simple exercise to help "let it go" and relax your system. Take very slow breaths, concentrating the breath into your lower belly. Begin to slowly breathe in the word "Let" through your nose. Exhale the word "go" slowly through your mouth. While you're doing this, allow everything in your body to relax and soften. Next, breathe in "I" and exhale "surrender," again softening and letting all your tension go as you exhale. Finally, breathe in "my" and exhale "body relaxes" as you completely relax and your shoulders drop, your jaw relaxes, and you unclench your bottom, legs, and stomach. Do this a minimum of 5 times.

This type of breathing exercise is great to practice now. This is one of my favorite breathing exercises, and I always do it with my clients in labor. The more relaxed you can help yourself become now, the more you'll be able to surrender to the process of labor in a few months.

FLAPPING FISH POSE

This pose encourages proper digestion and bowel movements, relaxes the nerves in your legs, and redistributes excess weight around your waistline. Many women experience pressure and blockage of circulation later in pregnancy, and this pose is great for women who are uncomfortable or who have trouble sleeping or relaxing. Here's how it works.

Lie on your right side with your hands under your cheek and your fingers interlocked.

Bend your left leg and bring your left knee up near your ribs. Keep your right leg straight.

While remaining lying down, slowly move your arms to the left until your left elbow is touching your left knee. Allow your arm to rest on the floor.

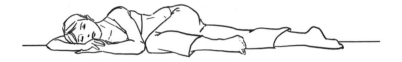

Rest your right cheek on your right arm.

Concentrate on your breathing and relax your entire body while feeling a gentle stretch.

Change sides.

If it helps, support your bent knee and head with pillows for extra comfort.

CHAIR POSE

Chair Pose provides a massage for the abdomen and digestive system.

Stand up straight with your feet together and your arms by your side.

Raise your arms shoulder-width apart with palms facing each other.

Keep stretching your arms and hands upward, and then slowly bend your knees as much as you can. As you bend your knees, your body and arms will naturally start to lean forward. Your knees and thighs should still be touching or as close together as possible.

While in this position, tilt your pelvic bone forward. This will feel like you're rounding your spine and creating a bit of a hollow in your abdomen.

Hold the pose for 30 seconds, breathing slowly and deeply.

Release the pose by slowly standing up straight and bringing your arms back down.

SUPPORTED BRIDGE POSE WITH BLOCK

The Supported Bridge Pose stretches the chest, neck, and spine; strengthens the legs; helps with digestion; calms the brain; and alleviates stress. When I have clients do this pose, I want to avoid any overstretching of the belly. I love doing a restorative version of the Bridge Pose by putting a block or a sturdy cushion under your sacrum (the spot right above the top of your butt) for support of your belly and back.

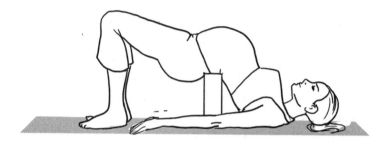

Lie on your back on a mat and bend your knees until your feet are flat on the floor and your heels are a few inches in front of your buttocks. Your knees should be lined up with your ankles and your feet parallel at hip-distance apart.

Put your arms on the floor at your sides. In order to practice a restorative version of the pose, place a yoga block under your sacrum (a spot you may have to play around to find, around the top of your buttocks). You can place the block at whatever level you feel is most comfortable. Place it on its highest level for the deepest opening of the pose.

Relax deeply in this version and let the block support your weight entirely. Close your eyes and enjoy.

To release the pose, lift up slightly on your toes as you remove the block from under your sacrum. Press your feet into the floor as you lower your hips back to the floor, one vertebra at a time. Try to keep this motion very controlled. Feel each section of your back gently return to the floor. Hug your knees toward your chest (making room for your belly, obviously) and rock side to side for a few counts to counteract the backbend.

ROCK THE SQUATS

Doing squats during pregnancy is great for a number of reasons, and not just to help relieve constipation. Squats help strengthen your legs and open and release tension in your hips, lower back, and feet. They can also prevent hemorrhoids and develop the flexibility a mom-to-be needs for giving birth in a natural posture. Squatting fully opens the birth canal, maximizes the power of the abdominal muscles, and helps protect the pelvic floor from injury.

Like Kegels, doing squats regularly will help keep your pelvic floor strong, even after pregnancy, so don't stop doing them postbirth. I recommend practicing squats as well as Kegels throughout your pregnancy; you can do them until the very end. If you are at risk for preterm labor, check with your caregiver about doing squats.

Here's a squat you can practice at any time during pregnancy.

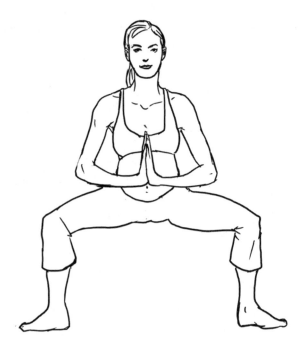

Get in a squatting position on a mat with your feet about shoulder-distance apart. Make sure your toes are pointed out and your heels are flat on the floor.

Give your belly plenty of space (especially during the later months of your pregnancy) by widening the space between your knees and separating your feet farther if necessary.

When in the squat position, bring your palms together in front of your chest (heart), so that your elbows push against the insides of your knees to intensify the opening of the hips. Stay here for 30 seconds to 1 minute and feel the stretch throughout your hips and back.

Try sitting on a folded blanket to feel the stretch without having to hold yourself up. You can also place a bolster or blocks under your pelvis to support your back. This is a great option toward the end of

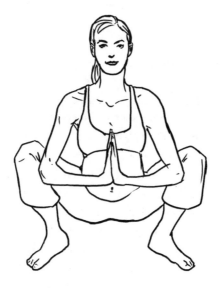

Ina May Gaskin, author of *Ina May's Guide to Childbirth* and a leading figure for midwives and doulas since the 1970s, has famously been quoted as saying, "Squat 300 times a day, you're going to give birth quickly."

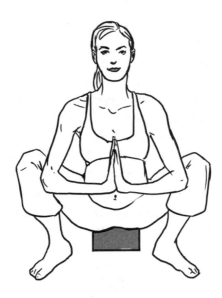

pregnancy when the weight of your body may be harder to support. Keep your elbows in position against your inner thighs in order to help your back remain straight and deepen the stretch.

Don't forget to breathe! You can even do a Kegel while squatting to connect with your pelvic floor. While inhaling, say the word "Let" as you pull your pelvic floor upward. Hold this position for 10 counts and say the word "go" as you exhale and unclench your vagina and butt as everything relaxes. This is good for body awareness, as you'll connect with the area of your body that will eventually help with pushing.

Come out of the pose the way that feels comfortable for you. The simplest and safest way to release a squat is to place your hands on the ground and use them for support as you straighten your legs and slowly come up to standing, one vertebrae at a time.

NATURAL REMEDIES FOR A CLEAR COMPLEXION

People speak of the "glow" many women have while pregnant. But if you're experiencing pregnancy-related acne, it can leave you feeling less than attractive, self-conscious, and stressed about your appearance. Some women experience acne from the very beginning of pregnancy. Others develop it later on, and some aren't affected by pregnancy acne at all. Why do some women get pregnancy acne while others don't? It usually has to do with their past history of acne. Chances are, if you had it earlier in life, you'll most likely get it again during pregnancy. Pregnancy acne is caused by an increase in hormone levels and the production of more oil that comes through the skin.

During this time, it's important to keep your skin clean. Here are some natural remedies I recommend to help keep pregnancy acne under control.

- Wash your face within 15 minutes of working out. This will clean the sweat and oil buildup from your workout off your skin and keep your pores clear.

- Certain natural elements can dry out pimples without using chemicals. These include lavender essential oil, lemon juice, toothpaste, aloe vera gel, plain yogurt, and tea tree oil.

- Use pure, organic coconut oil as a facial moisturizer. Coconut oil has antibacterial and antifungal properties to help prevent acne. Apply a thin layer to your face once a day or more. Replacing other cooking oils or butter with coconut oil can help benefit your skin and immune system, too.

- If you feel an outbreak coming on, ice your face for a few minutes to help reduce inflammation.

- Don't pick or pop pimples, as it might cause them to spread or scar.

- Avoid processed sugar, artificial sweeteners (which I hope you aren't using anyway), and white flour. What you're eating can directly affect how your skin looks and feels. Increasing greens and drinking more water can also help keep your skin healthy and cause fewer breakouts.

- Try not to wear makeup when you don't have to. Makeup can clog pores and increase oil, creating pimples. If you must wear makeup, try wearing oil-free or noncomedogenic makeup, which will avoid adding oils to your skin. Be sure to keep your makeup brushes clean, and wash your face as soon as you can, to let your skin breathe makeup-free.

- Use light, organic soap to wash your face. Harsh chemicals in many soaps strip your skin of necessary oils. If you get rid of all the oil on your face, it will only produce more. Wash your face gently. Don't scrub, and pat your skin dry with a clean towel.

Acne Mask

This is a great homemade pregnancy acne mask I use for my clients. The ingredients are easy to find and you can use it weekly to help relax the skin on your face and prevent further breakouts.

½ cup plain organic yogurt

1 tablespoon aloe vera gel

Juice of ¼ lemon

5 drops tea tree oil

In a bowl, combine the yogurt, aloe vera gel, lemon juice, and tea tree oil. Put the mixture on your entire face and leave it on for 10 minutes. Wash the mask off with warm water and pat your face dry.

YOGA FOR STRESS RELIEF

Start on the road to restfulness now. Try these yoga poses every day at home, and see how your mood—and your ability to sleep— will improve as your yoga practice becomes more consistent. The following exercise and poses are gentle and specifically designed to help you destress and decompress.

ALTERNATE NOSTRIL BREATHING EXERCISE

This is an amazing breathing exercise for stress relief, called *Nadi Shodhana*. In Sanskrit, *Nadi* means "channel" and *Shodhana* means "cleansing" or "purifying." In this exercise, you're going to clean and purify the channel of your nostrils, an essential part of your body that keeps breath flowing in and out of your body. By keeping your nostrils clear, your energy will flow clearly and the balanced oxygen flow to both sides of your brain will aid with stress relief and focus. Here's how it works.

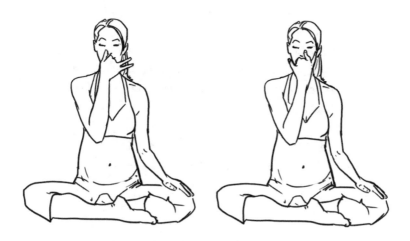

Sit in a comfortable, cross-legged position. You can sit on a folded blanket and support your back with a pillow, bolster, or yoga block. These aids can also be placed under your knees to reduce pressure. Sit up straight, but relax your body. Relax your jaw and face and breathe naturally.

(continued)

With your right hand, bend your index and middle fingers, keeping your ring finger, pinkie finger, and thumb extended.

Close your right nostril with your right thumb.

Inhale deeply through your left nostril.

When you can't inhale any deeper, close your left nostril with the ring finger of your right hand. Release your thumb from your right nostril and exhale through your right nostril.

Keeping the left nostril closed, inhale deeply through your right nostril.

Cover your right nostril again with your thumb, then release your left nostril.

Exhale out of your left nostril. You should now be in the original position, with your thumb sealing your right nostril. This is one cycle. Balance your inhalations and exhalations so they are the same length through both nostrils.

Breathe for a count of 4 to 6 for each breath, both as you inhale and exhale. Try to do 10 rounds of this breathing technique. It takes practice and patience, but once you get it down you'll find yourself taking time out to practice your alternate breathing technique wherever you are.

"If you want to conquer the anxiety of life, live in the moment, live in the breath."

—Amit Ray

Restorative Yoga Poses

Whether or not you already actively participate in yoga classes or do yoga at home, these restorative poses will help you do just what the name says—restore and revive your body, mind, and spirit. The following are gentle yoga poses that can be done any time of day when you want to relax and bring yourself back to center. One of the greatest benefits of these quieter yoga poses is that they offer you time—time to connect with and listen to your body and baby, and time to gain a better understanding of your own inner thoughts and feelings.

Some of the other benefits of restorative poses are that they:

- Reduce stress
- Reduce muscle tension
- Slow the heart rate
- Lower blood pressure
- Slow the breathing rate
- Increase bloodflow to major muscles
- Help concentration
- Calm and unplug the nervous system
- Help relieve insomnia and anxiety

CHILD'S POSE WITH BOLSTER

Relaxing in Child's Pose helps calm the mind, but as your belly gets bigger, you may need the extra support of a bolster or pillows.

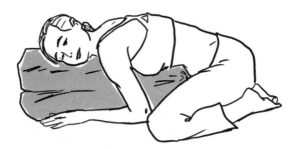

Start in a kneeling position and place a bolster or stack of pillows in front of you on the floor. Drop your butt toward your heels as you stretch the rest of your body down and forward, resting the front of your body on the bolster or pillows (making space for your belly between your legs, if needed).

Your arms should be in a relaxed position either along the floor or in front of you, hugging the pillows or bolster. Rest your forehead on the bolster or pillows and remain there as long as you need to.

SEATED CROSS-LEGGED FORWARD BEND WITH CHAIR

This pose releases lower back pain and hip tightness, combats fatigue and headaches, and helps calm the mind.

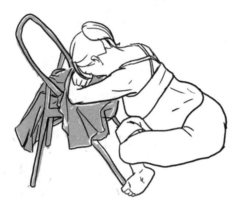

Place a chair facing you, and sit in a cross-legged position on the floor. Fold your body forward, resting your arms on the chair and resting your forehead on your forearms. Stay in that position as long as you need to.

RECLINED BOUND ANGLE POSE WITH BOLSTER

This pose can be deeply relaxing. It opens up your entire body and allows you to practice breathwork as well.

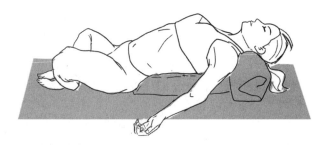

In a seated position, with your back to the bolster, bring the soles of your feet together and let your knees fall open to the sides (Butterfly Pose). Begin to recline back, making sure your lower back is up against the bolster. If this is too difficult, you can place two towels or yoga blankets under your knees for support. Place your arms out to the side, resting them on the floor, and practice the stress-relieving breathwork from earlier in this chapter.

YOGA POSES FOR ROUND LIGAMENT PAIN

If you're beginning to feel the effects of your uterus expanding to make room for baby, that means the lower part of your abdominal area—belly, pelvis, and groin—could be a little sore and achy. I talked about round ligament pain and ways to help relieve symptoms in the Your Changing Body section of this chapter. Here are some yoga poses you can do on a daily basis to help stretch your back and open up your pelvic area. By stretching your lower body, you'll feel less pain and be able to move a little easier.

CAT/COW POSE

Start on your hands and knees with your hands shoulder-distance apart and your knees hip-distance apart. As you inhale, look up while slowly arching your back and lifting your tailbone up to the sky. As you exhale, look down while rounding your back up and tucking your tailbone down toward the floor.

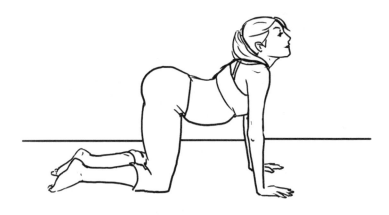

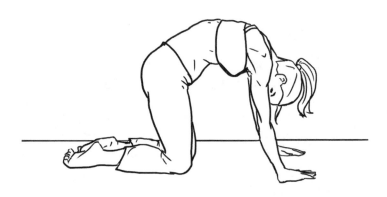

PUPPY DOG POSE

Start on your hands and knees with your hands shoulder-distance apart and your knees slightly wider than your hips. Slowly slide your hands forward, palms down, until you can place your forehead on the floor. At the same time, lift your butt in the air. Breathe deeply into your lower back and belly and stay here for five deep breaths. Feel the stretch in your spine. To release the pose, walk your arms slowly back toward your body, ending back on your hands and knees. Puppy Dog Pose is a close cousin of Downward-Facing Dog Pose. It's a good alternative if Downward-Facing Dog is too strenuous.

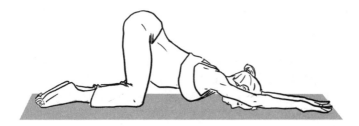

LOW LUNGE

The Low Lunge opens the hips and chest, stretches your groin and legs, and lengthens your spine.

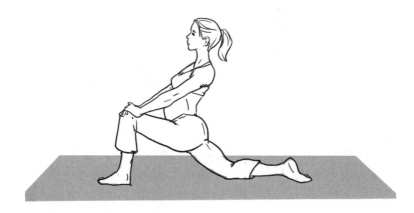

Start this pose by kneeling. Slide your left foot forward until your heel is flat on the ground and a little to the left (to help with your balance). Stretch forward until your left knee is directly over your left ankle. Place your hands on your knee, and make sure your back knee stays on the ground.

Hold this pose for three to six full breaths.

To release, inhale and slide your left leg forward, or step your right foot back and go into Downward-Facing Dog. Switch sides and repeat.

LIZARD POSE

Lizard Pose is a great hip opener, and it also stretches the hamstrings and thighs.

From Downward-Facing Dog, step your left foot forward, just outside of your left elbow, coming into a lunge.

Keep your hands on the mat, and stretch your right leg straight back behind you.

Keep your arms straight and press your chest forward. This will help encourage your hips to lower, increasing the stretch.

Look down at the floor and hold this pose for five breaths. Switch sides and repeat.

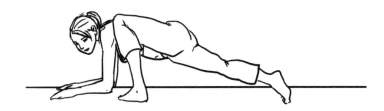

DESTRESS WITH TEA

Tea is amazing for your body during pregnancy. Herbal teas help with hydration and help lower stress levels. Many teas are high in antioxidants, can help with morning sickness, and prep your uterus for labor. There are always debates about what teas are safe for pregnant women to drink. Yes, there are certain herbal teas to avoid drinking, but there are so many more you can enjoy every day.

- Ginger tea eases nausea, helps with digestion, and relieves stomach issues. If you can't find ginger tea loose or in tea bags, add four or five slices of fresh ginger to boiled water and enjoy.
- Peppermint tea is great for settling an upset stomach, as well as helping with the nausea and vomiting common in early pregnancy.

DIY PREGNANCY TEA

- ½ cup loose dried red raspberry tea leaves
- ½ cup loose dried nettle tea leaves
- 2 tablespoons dried mint leaves
- 2 tablespoons dried alfalfa
- 2 tablespoons loose chamomile tea
- 2 tablespoons loose rose hip tea

In a bowl, mix together the raspberry and nettle tea leaves, mint leaves, alfalfa, chamomile tea, and rose hip tea. Store in an airtight container.

To serve, place one serving of the tea leaf mixture in a tea strainer or ball. Add to a cup of hot water and let the tea steep for a few minutes. Add honey and milk, if desired.

- Nettle tea provides high levels of iron, magnesium, and calcium, minerals all pregnant women need every day.
- Dandelion leaf tea is high in potassium and has a gentle but effective diuretic effect. Try adding dandelion leaf to another tea because it has a naturally grassy, bitter flavor.
- Rooibos tea is highly recommended in pregnancy. It's caffeine free and contains calcium, magnesium, and tons of antioxidants. It also has positive effects on digestion and can ease colic and reflux.
- Raspberry leaf tea prepares the uterus for labor and prevents postpartum hemorrhaging. It's also high in calcium and magnesium and is safe to drink from the second trimester onward.

TEAS TO AVOID DURING PREGNANCY

Many teas are considered unsafe during pregnancy because of their caffeine content, which is still a big debate. Research that spanned 10 years from the Norwegian Institute of Public Health suggests that caffeine consumption during pregnancy has been directly linked with reduced birth weights. However, the American College of Obstetricians and Gynecologists states that if you keep caffeine at 200 milligrams a day, your baby won't be negatively affected. You can always speak with your caregiver about caffeine, but I recommend that my clients try to avoid caffeine. Teas with high caffeine levels include:

- Black
- Green
- Oolong
- Lapsang souchong
- Hong Mao Feng
- Earl Grey
- Darjeeling

Other teas and herbs to avoid during pregnancy due to their risk of side effects include:

- St. John's wort
- Ginseng
- Yarrow
- Pennyroyal
- Ephedra
- Licorice root

There is still some discussion about how safe green tea is for pregnant women. Green tea can contain large amounts of caffeine and is said to reduce folic acid absorption.

Elissa Goodman's Iron Juice

My dear friend and holistic nutritionist Elissa Goodman swears by this blood-building juice. I have all my clients drink this during pregnancy and always after the birth.

2 beets, cut into chunks. Beets are a unique source of betaine, a nutrient that helps protects cells, proteins, and enzymes from environmental stress. They're also known to help fight inflammation, protect internal organs, boost stamina, and lower blood pressure.

6–8 kale leaves. Kale is great for cardiovascular support and is high in a ton of vitamins and minerals, including vitamins K (for bone health), A (for vision and skin), and C (for your immune system and metabolism).

Large handful of spinach. The folate in spinach helps prevent birth defects and protects against cell mutation. Spinach also helps build strong bones and teeth and lowers blood pressure (via its calcium and magnesium); is good for the lymphatic, urinary, and digestive systems; and has a laxative effect and is great for easing constipation. And it helps clear the body of toxins and is a blood builder, which means it's a great food to battle anemia.

2 oranges, peeled, sectioned, and seeded. Oranges are an amazing citrus fruit with many health benefits. The fiber in oranges helps prevent constipation, and their vitamin C works to prevent viral infections and heart disease. Oranges are also a lower-glycemic food, which means their natural sugars won't spike your blood sugar levels. They will also help your body absorb the iron from the vegetables in the juice.

Place the beets, kale, spinach, and oranges in a juicer. Juice and drink immediately.

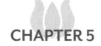

CHAPTER 5

Month Five

CULTIVATE YOUR INTUITION

"Trust yourself. You know more than you
think you do."

—**Benjamin Spock**

All women have motherly instincts—some just may not have
learned how to trust and follow them. The trick to tap into
your motherly intuition is to quiet the mind, let go of projections,
and learn to distinguish between the "fear voice" and your inner
knowing. Learning to trust and follow your gut takes time,
patience, and the wisdom that you already have the answers you
need to know within yourself. (You do!)

During your pregnancy and after the birth, you're going to get
a lot of opinions on what is right for you and your baby. Now is
the time to explore and make choices that feel right for *you*. Play

around with following your hunches, doing what feels right for you even if it might not make sense to others. If you don't trust your own intuition, you can easily be swayed and make important choices out of fear.

I used to teach a healing yoga class. Each week I would use a different theme and move that energy and suggestion through the body. One of my themes was connecting with and finding your inner guru. We all have one. It's that wise higher self that resides in each and every one of us. I know so many people who look outside themselves for all the answers—they search for the guru, teacher, doctor, or therapist who will tell them what to do, the best path for them to take. When you do this, you give away your power to make important choices and put it in someone else's hands. A good teacher will help point you in the right direction to find this power within, instead of looking outside for the answers. All you need to do is get quiet and still enough to listen and have the guts to follow what you hear, feel, or see even if it might not make sense.

> "When you don't know what to do, get still.
> The answer will come."
>
> —Oprah Winfrey

People search outside themselves for that special person, the guru who'll tell them what's best, when really, *each of us* is that person. You have all the answers within. When you can still your mind, you'll get in touch with that inner guru. This is where intuition is most important. See, intuition usually doesn't make sense until you follow it. It's an unexplained knowing, a feeling, sense, hunch, dream, vision, body sensation, or voice that is totally neutral and clear, isn't rational, and has no emotional charge. Learning to read and follow your intuition will help you make the right choices not only for your birth, your children, and your family, but also in your entire life.

I have a very strong spiritual belief that our children choose us before they are born. Before we are born, we all make a soul contract with our parents. It doesn't matter how your baby may come to you—if you carry him in your womb or use someone else's body, egg, or sperm. I believe even stepchildren are your destined children. Because of this contract, there is a deep knowing of one another from deep down in the depths of your soul. You have already met your baby, and if you trust that you already know each other on a soul level, then tuning in to your baby within will make it easier to connect with what he needs and who he is.

"Trust your hunches. They're usually based on facts filed away just below the conscious level."

—Dr. Joyce Brothers

When we don't trust our own internal knowing, we may let others sway us and make our decisions for us. I once worked with a client whose doctor kept pushing to induce labor early or perform a C-section because he was worried that her baby was going to be too big. She called me, saying, "I know my doctor wants me to do this but I *feel* that this baby isn't as big as they say and I will have a great birth." I asked her what made her feel this way. She explained, "It's this knowing I feel deep down in my core. If I just let things happen on their own, it will be fine. Even though I trust my doctor, I feel torn because I can't shake this feeling." I told her this was her gut knowing and to trust it. She talked with her doctor, who reluctantly went along with her wishes, and a few days after her estimated due date, she beautifully birthed a 7-pound baby boy with ease.

We place so much trust in medical doctors, but even they can't guarantee anything 100 percent. That's one of the reasons why it's so important to hone a mother's instinct. The hardest part about trusting your intuition is first finding out how your intuition speaks to you. I remember when I started playing around with finding my intuition. I was confused about what was my inner knowing, what was my logical mind, what was wishful thinking, and what was fear. As you play around with this, you will start to see that each one of these "voices" has a very different tone and feeling.

Intuition is an unexplained, unemotional, neutral knowing, feeling, or sensation—like an aha moment where you just know something that comes out of nowhere without explanation. Fear is different. Fear is highly charged with emotion and usually masks some kind of past wound or insecurity. The "fear voice" or "fear vision" can stop you from making a decision or can paralyze you, making it hard to move forward in your life.

Here's a great example: One of my clients wanted to give birth through a VBAC (vaginal birth after Caesarean). Her labor was a long journey. At one point, she started spinning with fear about hemorrhaging and dying. She had explained to me when I was prepping her for birth that she had a fear about dying because her brother had died a few years before.

I placed my hand on her heart and had her slowly breathe, inhaling the vision, words, or feeling of the way she wanted her birth to go and exhaling any fear, worry, or anxiety she was feeling. After a few minutes of this, she became calmer and more centered. I had her open her eyes and look into mine and I asked her to answer my question without overthinking—just answer me right away when I snap my fingers. I asked her, "Are you going to hemorrhage, is this really true?" She said, "No" and followed with, "and I'm not having a C-section either. I'm going to push this baby out with ease." An hour later, that's exactly what happened.

You know your fear voice is speaking when an emotional charge masks something deeper. With intuition, you just feel it. Next you must sort out the thinking, logical mind from the feeling, body-centered intuition. Our thoughts are not our intuition. Thoughts are what we consciously process through our minds, but to be intuitive you must get out of your mind and into your body. You have to be attuned to your body to access your intuition, since it comes through feelings and sensations.

"Good instincts usually tell you what to do long before your head has figured it out."

—**Michael Burke, organizational behaviorist, Tulane University**

YOUR CHANGING BODY

The fifth month of pregnancy is your halfway point, a huge milestone! All of the functions I described in the chapter on Month Four are still going strong in Month Five. Your circulation and blood production are still increasing, as are your hormones and lung capacity, and your uterus is still growing. Increased bloodflow can cause some unpleasant (but harmless) side effects, including nosebleeds and bleeding gums when you brush your teeth. Your breasts are still growing, and you may see some veins at the surface of your skin.

Your uterus may be expanding so much that your ligaments and skin are feeling the effects. Has your belly become itchy and tight feeling? If you haven't started using any creams or oils for relief, now is a great time. While you can't prevent your belly from growing, using creams will provide temporary relief from itchy skin.

Back pain may also start to be an issue during the fifth month. Since your belly is starting to protrude a lot more, your back is trying to compensate for the shift in weight. This is when I start doing back relief yoga with my clients (which I'll share with you later in the chapter). Other natural back relief remedies include the following:

- Practice good posture. If you keep yourself from slumping over, you won't feel the effects of the extra weight as much. Try to be conscious of how you're sitting. Keep your back as straight as possible (without straining), with your chest high and your heart out to the world. Keep your shoulders low and your neck relaxed. If you need to, sit with pillows behind you for comfort and support.

- Sleep on your side with a body pillow, or a few stacked pillows, between your legs. When you get out of bed, slowly roll out instead of going right from a sitting to a standing position.

- Don't twist your back. You'll need to start becoming super conscious about how you turn and move your body to pick things up. Bend with your knees instead of your back to avoid stressing your lower back.

- Prenatal massage will help all parts of your body, and your back is no exception. Even though you can't lie on your stomach for a massage, a good massage therapist knows how to maneuver your back for relief or can use a pregnancy massage pillow or table.
- Start seeing a chiropractor.

One thing I stress to my clients is to keep exercising at this point, as long as you're having a healthy pregnancy. If you're uncomfortable, honor where you're at and back off or modify your exercise pace. If you are feeling great and strong, by all means continue your exercise routine. The benefits are priceless. Try walking more instead of jogging, or riding a recumbent stationary bike. Movement is so valuable for you and your baby-to-be.

YOUR GROWING BABY

Have you had your midpoint ultrasound yet? By now, you may have witnessed the absolutely amazing technology that helps you see your baby and all her parts. If you find out your baby's gender, you may even start referring to the baby as "he" or "she." Month Five involves a lot of development focusing on baby's protection. Fat, specifically a layer of brown fat, is developing under her skin. Although more layers of fat will form, this first one will be baby's best defense against the extreme temperature change she'll experience after birth. Three layers of skin that will create the best protection for baby are actually being created this month: the epidermis (outermost layer); dermis (middle layer); and subcutis (deepest layer, which is mostly the brown fat).

This is also the month that the coating called vernix caseosa (or just vernix) will start forming a protective layer outside your baby's skin. This is the white, slippery coating that looks milky or cheesy right when a baby is born. Vernix plays an essential role in keeping the fine outer layer of baby's skin from becoming chapped in the womb, and it also protects the soft lanugo (downy body hair) that's been growing as well.

Vernix has tons of great healing properties. This amazing substance acts as a deep moisturizer for baby's skin, helps to regulate baby's body temperature, and carries tons of antibacterial properties. This magical substance needs time to be fully absorbed into the skin. Instead of wiping it off right after birth, consider asking the birthing staff to leave it on your baby. It's most effective to wait 24 hours after birth before giving your baby a bath.

Finally, the bones that have been forming as tissue and marrow will start the process of ossification, or hardening. The legs and inner ear bones are the first to ossify, so it's no wonder that this is the time when you'll start to feel tiny butterfly kicks from your little one. His ears are going to be put to work, too. He can hear your blood pumping, your heart beating, your voice speaking, and even your stomach growling. These are all soothing sounds to your baby, and that may be one reason why newborns benefit from lying near your heart after birth—it brings them back to their comfort zone.

For the first time, your baby will be large enough to be measured from head to heel. By the end of the month, your baby will be around 6½ inches long (the length of a large banana) and will weigh around ½ pound.

During the second half of pregnancy, your baby will pee about 1 liter a day. Where does it go? They swallow it! But don't worry, it's perfectly natural and not harmful to them.

JOURNAL WORK: WATCHING AND LISTING THE THREE VOICES

"At times you have to leave the city of your comfort and go into the wilderness of your intuition. What you'll discover will be wonderful. What you'll discover is yourself."

—Alan Alda

Let's try an exercise to help you begin your practice of finding your intuition. Like I said before, it can be very difficult to distinguish between the three voices.

Intuition is an unexplained, neutral knowing, feeling, sensation, or flash of insight like an aha moment where you "just know" without explanation.

Fear is highly charged with emotion and usually masks some kind of past wound or insecurity. The fear voice or vision can be upsetting.

Thinking is mental chatter, thoughts, and processing.

For this next month, start to pay attention to the different voices, feelings, or sensations in your body and mind when making decisions about your pregnancy. Create three columns and write down the headings "Intuition," "Fear," and "Thinking." It's hard to know which voice is which if you aren't fully conscious of them, so writing down your thoughts and feelings about decisions you need to make, how you feel during conversations with your doctor or your partner, etc., will allow you to attribute your reactions to one of the voices.

Practice this exercise with your partner. Have her ask you a few simple questions and snap her fingers right away after asking each question. If you don't answer right when she snaps, have her move on to the next question. You will have already moved into thinking mode.

Start with some easy questions, like these:

● What's your favorite color?

- What's your favorite food?
- What's your favorite city?

Then, move on to some possibly unknown questions:

- What is the sex of your baby?
- What is his or her name?
- What does your baby need from you?

This "answering without thinking" exercise forces your intuition to take over. Some of it won't make any sense to you. For example, you might blurt out a totally off-the-wall name for your baby. I did this once with a client for fun. She responded that her baby was a boy and blurted out that his name was Gary. She was less than impressed with the name, but the letter G did resonate with her. It turned out that her dad, who had passed away, was named Gab, and she ended up naming her son Gabriel, after him. You never know where your spontaneous answering will lead! It may seem silly at first, but it can put you on the right path.

I once had a client with fertility issues. No matter what she tried, she couldn't get pregnant. She was a healthy, active woman who was ready to bring a baby into her home. We did some intuition work together, and during one exercise she was able to see her baby. She said he was a boy, his name was Liam, and he looked like a combination of her two brothers. When she asked what he needed from her to be born, she heard that he didn't want to be born into chaos.

She opened her eyes immediately and was shocked at what she'd heard and felt. She knew there was truth to it and understood that she needed to tweak some things in her life in order for him to come to her. We talked about what she could do to have a more calm, peaceful, and drama-free life. We did weekly coaching to work on her emotions dealing with her infertility and boundaries with family. She did yoga and massage to relax. She was also living in a temporary house as she renovated her home, so she worked hard to get her house in order so she could feel more settled. Well, 3 months after she moved into her new place, she got pregnant with a little boy she named Liam who, of course, looked just like her brothers.

BOND WITH YOUR BABY
THROUGH MUSIC AND YOUR VOICE

One great way to jump-start your motherly intuition is to lock in a few soothing tools to help you transition into parenthood and your baby transition into the world. You can start now with just the sound of your voice. Your voice will be the most familiar thing to your baby, so any way you can direct your voice to her will help the two of you bond.

Around the fifth month of pregnancy, I have my clients put together a playlist for their little one. These can be lullabies you love or grew up with or songs you and your partner like or that have a special meaning. I suggest playing music to your baby every night when you're relaxing. Try using headphones like Bellybuds on your belly. While the choice is ultimately yours, I do recommend avoiding anything too loud or jarring. Playing music to your baby nightly will make her become familiar with these songs. You can even play this mix during birth, and afterward use the playlist to soothe your baby during the day or at bedtime. This music will be familiar to her and will help with the transition from your womb into this world.

You can also try singing to your belly. If you don't know a good song, hum a tune or make one up. And don't worry: Your baby doesn't know—or care—if you have a good singing voice.

You can also read a few of your favorite children's books. I happen to love all of the inspirational ones out there, but feel free to read anything you love and want your baby to know. Both you and your partner can read the books out loud, so by the time you're 7 months pregnant, your baby will recognize your voices. As with playing music, reading books to your baby as she grows will make her familiar with them, and she will know the story by the reading tone you use.

These days, many fortunate people who wouldn't be able to have a child otherwise are able to have surrogates carry their babies for them. These folks can still do all of the above by making a recording for their baby-to-be. Have your surrogate play the sound of your voice daily to her belly. I did this with a few of my clients who used surrogates, and even a few who adopted. It was beyond helpful and healing to have familiar, soothing sounds for the parents and baby.

CONNECTING WITH YOUR BABY'S ENERGY: WRITE AN "I FEEL YOU" INTUITIVE LETTER

"Intuition is seeing with the soul."

—Dean Koontz

Get into a comfortable seated or lying position. Begin to breathe deeply into your heart, feeling and listening to your own heartbeat and the rhythm of your breath. When thoughts arise, notice them and label them as "thinking" and bring your attention back to your heart and breath. Do this for a few minutes until you're fully relaxed.

Next, send that breath deep into your baby in your belly. As you inhale, send your breath and life force into him. As you exhale, feel his energy inside you expanding, projecting further out into the world each time. Keep doing this for a few minutes. Sometimes at this point a vision or flash of a baby pops up. If you get one, remember what you saw, heard, or felt. If not, then with the next breaths call in your baby. Tell him to come to you and show himself to you. If you don't see anything, just breathe in these questions and keep feeling your baby's energy expand outward.

- Are you a boy or a girl?
- Is there anything you need?
- What do you look like?
- What's your energy like?
- Do you have a name, or what would you like us to call you?

Allow some time between questions to receive your baby's message. Focus on breathing into your belly and, as you exhale, concentrate on expanding your baby's energy out. Notice what you feel—again, intuition is a flash, hunch, feeling, or sense. Even if it comes in the form of a voice, it will just pop into your head.

Trust what you get and follow it. For example, if your baby needs peace, maybe do some things to relax and destress. If you hear the word *broccoli*—like one of my soon-to-be mamas did—then, by all means, go eat some broccoli. One of my clients saw her baby and had this overwhelming feeling in her heart when she asked what he needed from her that he wanted her and his dad to have peace in their relationship. They had been going through a rough patch the last 3 months of her pregnancy. She began crying and soon afterward started couples counseling with her husband.

If something isn't clear, ask for more clarity. Sometimes you might not get the answer right away. It might come to you in a dream or while you are at yoga or working out. (I get a lot of my answers while driving.) Practice tuning in daily, and you will be tapping into your baby in no time.

Don't get discouraged if you don't "get anything" right away. As with anything new, you need time and practice playing around to get good at it. On a piece of paper, jot down what you saw, heard, or felt—even if it sounds crazy. For fun, write a letter to your baby after tuning in to him. Write about what you saw, heard, and felt or just have a hunch about his energy, and what you sense he'll look and act like. If you really listen, you'll be surprisingly accurate.

INTUITIVELY NAMING YOUR BABY

Speaking of names, you can pick your baby's name by tuning in to its energy. It always amazes me when I get my clients calm and relaxed, have them close their eyes, and have them tell me, without thinking, what they feel this baby of theirs will look and act like. One hundred percent of the time they totally describe their child. I am always blown away by how accurate they were when I visit down the road.

Have you ever noticed that many people's names come with a certain energy? Emma, Grace, Rose, and Sophia are very feminine. Ace and Rocco have the energy of the tough guy, while Milo and Gabriel are softer. Lucy, Phoebe, Scarlett, and Ruby—you can just tell they're going to have some sass to them! After I have my clients connect with their baby, they usually say "He feels like a _____ (name)" or "She is a little lady," "She seems wise beyond her years," or that a "more traditional name" is a better fit for their child's energy.

If names aren't coming to you clearly yet, meditate on it and keep asking. You might have to wait to birth your baby to lock in the name, but trust that the name that pops into your head will be the right one. Also, telling people the name of your baby in advance can be tricky—you may get reactions that make you question your choice. I always suggest keeping your baby's name to yourself or sharing it with a few trusted people.

"Your inner knowing is your only true compass."

—Joy Page

When women from the Himba tribe of Namibia, Africa, know they are pregnant, they go out into the wilderness with other women and sing, chant, and meditate until they hear the "song" of the child. They believe that every soul has its own vibration that expresses its unique identity. When the women intuitively understand the song, they sing it out loud. They return to the tribe and teach it to everyone else in preparation for the baby's arrival. When the baby is born, the women of the tribe sing the song to the child. The song is also sung at different milestones, including each birthday, significant events, and when the child passes from the world.

YOGA FOR BACK PAIN

Earlier, I wrote about how back pain may become a regular occurrence for you around Month Five. Your belly is starting to grow, and the weight and imbalance of your body may take its toll on your back. Here are six simple yoga poses you can do daily to help with back pain. They will gently stretch your back without straining it, preparing your body for the day.

RESTORATIVE DOWNWARD-FACING DOG POSE

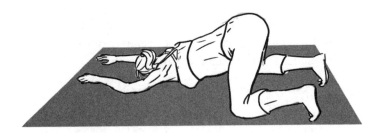

Start on your mat on all fours. Tuck your toes under and bring your heels up, lift your butt up, and press it back toward your heels. Reach your arms straight ahead of you, pressing your forehead onto the floor. Take a deep breath into your upper back through your nose and, as you exhale, allow your chest to drop.

CAT/COW POSE

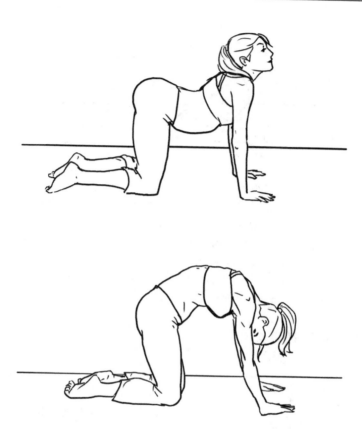

I introduced this pose earlier, but this is also a great pose to help with back pain. Again, start on all fours on your mat. Inhale deeply into your baby/belly as you arch your back (bring your head and tail-bone up). When you exhale, round your back (bring your head and tailbone down). Try to make each inhalation and exhalation last at least 4 counts, and slowly move your body with your breath.

HIP CIRCLES

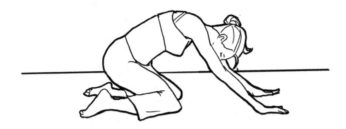

Still on all fours, begin to slowly make circles with your hips. After a few seconds, switch directions. You can also try Standing Hip Circles. Stand with your feet hip-width apart or wider and place your hands on your hips. Inhale and gently allow your pelvis to circle forward. Exhale and release your pelvis back to its original position. Allow your breath to guide the movement. When you complete a few circles in one direction, switch directions.

WAG THE TAIL

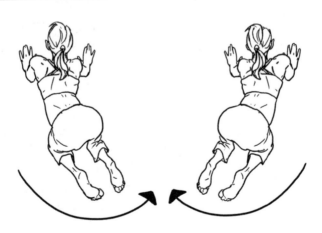

On all fours, slowly sway your hips from side to side like you're rocking your baby in a cradle.

SIDE STRETCH

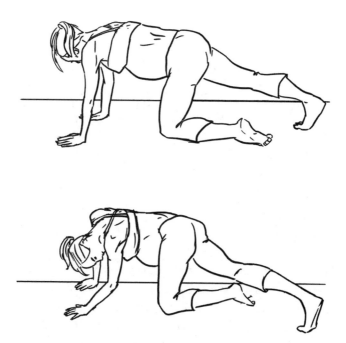

Get on all fours. Extend your right leg and gently swing it behind you over your left leg. Bend your elbows slightly and look behind you at your right foot. Take a deep breath into the side of your body and, as you exhale, let go of everything and relax. Switch sides to stretch your left side.

SEATED FORWARD BEND WITH CHAIR

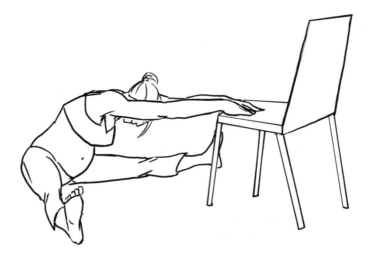

Sit on the floor with the seat of the chair facing you and your legs open straight out to the sides as far as they will go. Flex your feet so your toes are pointed toward the ceiling. Stretch your lower back and raise your arms above your head. Slowly reach and fall forward, keeping your spine straight. Place your hands on the seat of the chair in front of you. Hold for a few breaths while breathing deeply into your lower back.

PREGNANCY AND MUSCLE CRAMPS

One very common ailment during pregnancy is muscle cramping. Cramping in the feet, calves, or upper legs can happen when you least expect it. Have you ever woken up in the middle of the night with your calf cramping and on fire? Charley horses, which affect the calf muscles, can be painful. Muscle spasms occur mainly in the foot and calf muscles but can also happen in your entire leg, hands, arms, stomach, and rib cage.

Muscle cramps can have many possible causes. They include:

- Poor blood circulation in the legs
- Lack of exercise
- Overexertion of calf muscles
- Failure to stretch properly before exercise
- Muscle fatigue
- Dehydration
- Magnesium and/or potassium deficiency
- Calcium deficiency
- Lack of salt in the diet

There are many ways to help prevent and alleviate muscle cramps throughout pregnancy, including the following:

- Eat more foods high in vitamins and magnesium, potassium, and calcium. For more magnesium, eat bananas, brown rice, beans and lentils, raw spinach, and even a little dark chocolate. Potassium-rich foods include white beans, dark green leafy vegetables such as kale or spinach, acorn squash, sweet potatoes, dried apricots, bananas, avocados, asparagus, and zucchini. Calcium-rich foods include dairy products such as low-fat yogurt, cheese, and milk; tofu and soybeans; and broccoli and almonds.
- Try fortified cereals such as Total, raisin bran, and cornflakes. (They have a lot of calcium in one serving.)
- Drink fortified orange juice or soy milk.
- Stay well hydrated. (See my tips in Chapter 1.)
- Salt your food with Himalayan sea salt.
- Drink nettle leaf tea, which is high in calcium.
- Down a Natural Calm powdered drink before bed. (Buy the one with added calcium.)
- Massage your legs before bed with some arnica oil and a few drops of chamomile oil and lavender oil. You can also spray diluted magnesium oil on an area that has spasms. Dilute the

oil in a base such as coconut, almond, or jojoba oil, then massage it into your skin. The product called Ancient Minerals Magnesium Oil is great for this.

- Eat kelp or take kelp pills. Kelp is naturally high in potassium and iron, so it's great to help with anemia, too.

- Stretch properly before exercising.

- Get a full-body massage. Be sure to tell the masseuse to target areas that tend to cramp.

- Try my natural sports drink: coconut water with a packet of orange-flavored Emergen-C and a pinch of Himalayan sea salt.

- Elevate your legs for 10 to 20 minutes a day to improve circulation.

- Exercise often; it doesn't need to be strenuous. Walking, swimming, and yoga can all help stretch your leg muscles and prevent cramps.

- Apply warm, moist heat—a hot water bottle or heating pad—to your feet, calves, or other areas that tend to cramp. Muscle cramping responds well to heat.

- Wear socks to keep your feet warm. Try wearing socks that cover your calves to keep your muscles warm and prevent cramping.

- Eat one or two pickles. The high salt content will quickly replace the sodium you may have lost and will prevent cramping.

- Sleep on your left side. The vena cava, the large vein that brings unoxygenated blood to your heart, circulates blood to the left side of your body and your uterus. Lying on your left side will increase the blood and nutrients that reach the placenta.

- Drink 3 tablespoons of apple cider vinegar in ½ cup of orange juice at bedtime. Leg cramps can often be a sign that you're low in potassium, and apple cider vinegar is high in potassium.

- Drink tonic water with lemon. Tonic water contains quinine, and quinine has been shown to alleviate charley horses.

- Use ginger to help relieve muscle spasms. For a foot cramp soak, fill up a large pot with very warm water. Add 2 table-spoons of freshly grated ginger and 1 cup of Epsom salts, and soak for 10 minutes.
- Avoid wearing high heels.
- Avoid crossing your legs.
- Wear support hose during the day.
- Add ¾ cup of magnesium oil and 1¼ cups of Epsom salts to a warm bath. You can also add a few drops of lavender oil.
- Sleep with loose covers or blankets. Tightly tucked covers can press down your toes, possibly causing your calf and foot muscles to tighten and cramp. *The Complete Home Wellness Handbook* by Dr. John Swartzberg, Dr. Sheldon Margen, and the editors of the *UC Berkeley Wellness Letter* recommends sleeping on your side with your knees bent or loosening the sheets and blankets to keep them from weighing down your feet.

Even though they may not have science behind them, old wives' tales often work. Here are a couple of old wives' tales about leg cramps: Some people swear that placing a bar of lavender soap under the bed or under the bottom sheet will ward off leg cramps. Also, try placing a spoon by your bedside (it doesn't have to be silver; stainless steel is fine). When you awaken with a leg cramp, put the spoon on the cramp and it will uncramp instantly. Try it—you never know!

STRETCHES BEFORE BED

These are great, easy poses to stretch your legs and help with circulation.

STANDING CALF STRETCH

Stand facing a wall and extend one leg back. Lean toward the wall, pressing your back heel down until you feel tension in that leg. Hold the stretch for several seconds. Repeat on the other side. You can also do Downward-Facing Dog at the wall, alternately pressing each heel down to the floor.

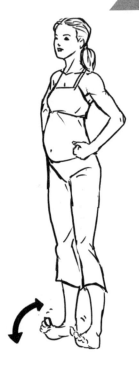

FIRE UP THE SHINS

Stand with both feet flat on the floor. Leaving your heels on the floor, lift all your toes up toward your head. Release and lower all your toes down quickly. Next, alternate your feet, tapping your toes up and down quickly 8 to 10 times.

QUADS STRETCH

Face a wall, and lean into it for support. Bend your left leg, bringing your heel toward your butt and keeping your knees together. Grab your left foot with your left hand. Hold for a few seconds, then switch sides.

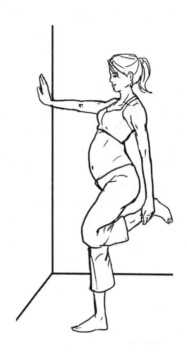

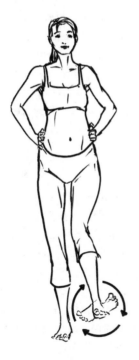

ANKLE ROLLS

Place your hands on your hips or use the wall for support, and lift your right leg off the floor a few inches. Slowly roll your right foot clockwise in a circle, then counterclockwise a few times. Switch legs and repeat.

INTUITIVE EATING

"Trust your gut."

—Unknown

In Chapter 1, I talked a lot about the right foods for fuel and nourishment. You may be a healthy eater already, or it may take practice to pin down the right foods for you on your food journey. For years, I followed certain diets and eating programs, thinking there was one right way for me to eat. From being vegan to following the raw diet, the Zone diet—you name it, I've tried it. I found the best way to eat by using my intuition. For me, following a strict eating program is too limiting, since my body needs different things at different times. Your body will tell you what it needs if you listen closely.

Women are very sensitive to smells during pregnancy. Amazingly, this is the mom-to-be's way of staying away from certain foods that might be harmful to her baby. A study in the journal *Behavioral and Neural Processes* explains how this sensitivity helps pregnant mothers avoid eating small levels of toxins that might not be dangerous to an adult but could be harmful to a fetus. For example, the smells of smoke, alcohol, and coffee are all particularly noticeable to pregnant women.

For this month, play around with your cravings and what your body is telling you. Forget the dieting mind-set or the idea that your food needs to be a certain way. Trust your body—you can also tune in to your baby and ask what she needs. If you crave something, research the benefits and healing qualities of the food.

Another simple thing to do before a meal is to ask yourself what you need and see what pops into your head. Foods like pizza or macaroni and cheese are comfort foods that might mean you need to nurture yourself and do some self-soothing. Craving empty calories that just fill you up, like popcorn or chips, might mean you are trying to stuff down an emotion. So what are you not allowing yourself to feel?

Jenna's Gluten-Free Pregnancy Pancakes

I first worked with Jenna when she was pregnant with her son and I've helped her through two pregnancies. She invented this pancake recipe and, needless to say, I went nuts over these. They're great for pregnancy because they're high in protein, omegas, and calcium. They also freeze well to keep on hand for a simple breakfast or snack.

6 cups gluten-free baking and pancake mix

¼ cup ground flaxseeds

1 container (16 ounces) organic cottage cheese

8 ounces Fage Total or 2% yogurt

5 eggs (I use 3 eggs and 5 egg whites)

2½ cups freshly squeezed orange or tangerine juice (or use almond milk or a mixture of half almond milk and half juice)

1½ teaspoons vanilla extract

Blueberries, chopped bananas, or chocolate chips (your choice)

Canola oil

Pure maple syrup (optional)

In a large bowl, mix together the baking mix, flaxseeds, cottage cheese, yogurt, eggs, juice, vanilla, and blueberries, bananas, or chocolate chips.

Heat some canola oil in a skillet. Use a ¼-cup measuring cup to scoop each pancake onto the skillet. Cook until the batter is just dry, 2 to 3 minutes per side. Top with pure maple syrup (or leave plain) and enjoy.

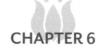

CHAPTER 6

Month Six

PATCH IT UP

"Let's raise children who won't have to recover from their childhoods."

—Pam Leo

There are many ways life experiences affect people as they grow. Both positive and negative experiences shape us from the very beginning of life. Some moments stay in the forefront of memory, while others are pushed back and forgotten. Unfortunately, some events from our past might have wounded us. These wounds can come back and haunt us during adulthood. They can often be triggered when you're about to have children of your own or even when you're already a parent. The resurfacing of past wounds can affect not only your quality of life but also that of your friends, family, and, most important, your children. This energy you carry within is what therapists refer to as your *wounded or hurt inner child*.

What is your inner child, anyway? The inner child is the childlike aspect of our selves, including all we learned and experienced as children. We were all children once, and we still have that child dwelling within us. Most adults, however, are unaware of this.

The definition of a *wounded* inner child goes beyond the idea that we all still have a child within us who needs to be heard, nurtured, and expressed. John Bradshaw, an educator and popular psychology and self-help movement leader, famously used the phrase *inner child* to point to unresolved, wounding childhood experiences and the lingering dysfunctional effects of childhood. Bradshaw's definition of inner child refers to the sum total of mental-emotional memories stored in the subconscious from conception through prepuberty.

Thich Nhat Hanh, one of the world's leading teachers of mindfulness and meditation, describes the concept of the inner child this way: "In each of us, there is a young, suffering child. We have all had times of difficulty as children and many of us have experienced trauma. To protect and defend ourselves against future suffering, we often try to forget those painful times. Every time we're in touch with the experience of suffering, we believe we can't bear it, and we stuff our feelings and memories deep down in our unconscious mind. It may be that we haven't dared to face this child for many decades."

The inner child is the lost, frightened, or forgotten child within. Some adults prefer not to remember painful childhood suffering, so they block it out or stuff the memories deep down within. The pain is always there, however, lurking around to come back out and affect their lives and those around them when they least expect it. It's like sweeping dirt under a carpet; eventually, the dirt has nowhere to go but *out*. This child within needs and wants to be let out, heard, nurtured, and have its needs met.

The trick to establishing a better relationship with your inner child? Have that child *speak* to you, not act out in the world. We can do that by actually working on developing a relationship with and integrating those wounded or forgotten parts of ourselves.

JOURNAL WORK

"Before I fix the world, I have to fix myself."

—Evan Meekins, *The Black Banner*

This month, I want to help you start to find ways to calmly and effectively patch up issues within yourself. These can include not getting the love and nurturing you needed as a child; abandonment issues; not being accepted for who you are; or being smothered and controlled by an overbearing parent. These are not the most comfortable or pleasant topics to deal with, but they are also things you don't want to repeat with or put on your own children.

Since this chapter talks about your inner child and patching things up with family, friends, and yourself, I have a few writing exercises to explore different sides of your childhood.

- Make a list of your own misbehaviors, unmet needs, disappointments, or past hurts as a child. How can you help nurture and parent your inner child today?

- What are the sacred things from your past that you want to keep alive and bring into your new family? Write out all of your positive experiences and memories from your childhood. These can include family traditions, rituals, and values that you want to keep and pass on wholeheartedly to your child.

- Make a list of all the qualities you love about your partner and her strengths. You can use these to be better parents. For example, if one of you is more nurturing and the other is better with discipline, you can find the balance in your roles *before* your baby is born.

We must find the courage to heal this part of ourselves, not only to live more fully, but also for the benefit of our children and all those around us, as well.

When people begin to raise a child, the wounded inner child can often get in the way of successful parenting. They either repeat the wounding they experienced in childhood or become the polar opposite of how their own parents acted during their childhood. Children are born with their own path to walk, and their parents' wounds are not for them to carry. However, you also can't heal what you aren't aware of.

"Every child is an artist. The problem is how to remain an artist once he grows up."

—Pablo Picasso

I have seen overbearing parents smothering their children because they themselves never received the love they needed. Instead of learning to find that love within, they look for their children or others or things to fill that void. This is way too much pressure and responsibility to put on another person, much less a child. When you look outside yourself to fill the void of emptiness or loneliness, you will be fulfilled—temporarily. In time, it won't be enough because the only one that can truly fill that void is you.

YOUR CHANGING BODY

In the sixth month of pregnancy, there's no denying that you're pregnant. Every woman is different, and there's no telling how small or large your belly will look as your pregnancy progresses. Your uterus is now around 1½ to 2½ inches above your belly button and the size of a basketball. You may start comparing yourself to other pregnant women. Pregnant bellies come in all different shapes and sizes. No matter what your size, I hope you're connecting with the miracle of making a baby and celebrating your beautiful shape and the amazing work your body is doing.

Up until around Month Six, your levels of the hormones progesterone and estrogen have been pretty similar, with progesterone slightly higher. This month, it's estrogen's turn to catch up and then surpass progesterone production. This could create a surge in emotions you haven't experienced since the first trimester.

Your rib cage is also beginning to expand, due to the increase in oxygen reaching your lungs. You can't feel this shift in your chest, but you may start to (or continue to) experience shortness of breath during this time. Your baby is large enough to crowd the space near your ribs, which can cause discomfort and shortness of breath. This isn't baby's permanent position, however: Before you give birth, your little one will begin to drop into your pelvic area.

You're not completely down the homestretch of pregnancy just yet, but your uterus is ready to warm up for labor. It's totally possible to begin feeling what's called Braxton Hicks contractions. These are generally mild, inconsistent feelings of your belly quickly tightening and relaxing. They last only a few seconds and shouldn't be painful. Braxton Hicks contractions are called "practice contractions" because it's your uterus getting ready for the big day. They are not dangerous for you or your baby. Here are some differences between Braxton Hicks contractions and regular labor contractions.

- Braxton Hicks contractions are concentrated in one area of your belly, while regular labor moves throughout your belly and lower back.

- Braxton Hicks contractions don't affect any other part of your body. With true labor, your cervix begins to dilate as well.

- Finally, Braxton Hicks contractions come infrequently. True labor is more frequent, has a consistent pattern to it that doesn't go away, and can come with a cramping feeling. As always, if you're not sure what you're feeling, call your caregiver.

Feeling tired and irritable? Eat a banana! Bananas contain serotonin and tryptophan, natural mood enhancers that relax the mind as well as provide a good source of natural energy.

Aside from possible practice contractions, you're also likely feeling your baby kick more, since he's getting stronger and he still has plenty of room in there to play around. You may even feel some quick, hiccuplike bumps coming from your belly. Don't worry about those, either, because that's your baby actually hiccupping. He is starting to swallow, so fluid and oxygen carried from your placenta can cause bubbles in his own little belly.

Did you know that all the eggs you will ever produce in your lifetime are stored in your ovaries before you are born?

YOUR GROWING BABY

It's all about the lungs this month. Hearing a newborn cry for the first time after birth is one of the most joyous, welcome sounds you'll ever experience. A baby taking its first breath is an announcement to the world that she has arrived. Your baby's lungs are preparing for the outside world in multiple ways. First, the substance called surfactant is beginning to do its job. Surfactant lines the air sacs in the lungs to help them easily inflate and deflate without sticking together or collapsing. The blood vessels in the lungs are also growing and strengthening, allowing your baby to take little "breaths" for the first time. Of course, your baby's lungs are still filled with fluid, but practice makes perfect.

Finally, your baby is starting to experience two other senses—taste and touch. Taste buds are beginning to form on her tiny tongue. Your baby's brain and nerve ends are also working together well enough to recognize sensations on her fingertips. Of course, she's not "touching" anything in particular, but this is the time when you may see your baby on an ultrasound sucking her thumb or putting her hands on her face.

By the end of the sixth month, the average baby measures around 10 inches long and weighs about 12 ounces. She is about the length and weight of an average ear of corn.

PARTNER UP

*"The most important thing a father can do for
his children is to love their mother."*

—Rev. Theodore Hesburgh

I've heard many times from clients and friends that "maybe when we have a child our relationship will get better." I hate to be the bearer of bad news, but if there are problems in your relationship before a child comes into your world, having a baby will only add salt to the wound. It's really important to patch up

TRAVELING WHILE PREGNANT

Thinking of going on a "babymoon" vacation before your baby arrives? If you're flying or going on a long car ride to get to your destination, be very aware of maintaining circulation in your legs. I always suggest wearing compression stockings when traveling, both during and after a flight or car ride. Compression stockings will help keep circulation flowing and prevent swelling, blood clots, and varicose veins.

Most caregivers advise against traveling after Month Seven or Eight (depending on your caregiver and whether you have a high-risk pregnancy or are at risk for preterm labor).

Here are more tips for a comfortable travel experience.

- Put your legs up throughout the flight.
- Get up and walk around every hour.
- Do ankle rolls, and flex and point your feet.
- Wear loose, comfortable clothing.
- Drink tons of water to stay extra hydrated.
- Take your shoes off during a flight or car ride.

your relationships and get on the same page as your partner before having children. Or start working together as quickly as possible once you discover you are pregnant. Babies may be temporary fixes, but they don't solve bigger problems.

Children see and pick up on *everything*. We don't give them enough credit for the things they are aware of. They're sensitive to the energy surrounding them. Even though you might not openly fight with your partner, children can feel subtle negative energy. They can sense the tension, resentment, and anger. No relationship is perfect, and even the very best relationships have their ups and downs. What I'm talking about is the overall state of a relationship. It's like the 70/30 rule: What you do 70 percent of the time is what makes the biggest impact on your life.

While I do occasionally see couples whose relationships are strained during my time working with them, I'm also blessed to work with many couples who are positive role models. These couples demonstrate what a positive and healthy relationship is, and I can clearly see how their children thrive from it. I've asked all of these different couples that I respect and admire what they do to have what they have with each other. I find it interesting that they've all said these things.

1. We want each other to be happy, and we do what we can to make this happen.

2. We have a deep love and respect for each other.

3. We are supportive of each other.

Here's a great example: I worked with a husband and wife who had a wonderfully mindful relationship. They read a book called *Brain Rules for Baby* by John Medina, and they especially loved the relationship chapter in the book, which discussed four things that cause postbaby conflicts in relationships: sleep loss, social isolation, unequal workloads, and depression. This couple was mindfully empathetic and committed to having each other's back by noticing when the other might need more sleep, need to get out of the house, or be feeling a bit blue and need extra attention to lift his or her spirits. He might have said, "You seem a little tired. Why don't you go take a nap and I'll take the baby to the park?" Or, if he seemed antsy and irritable, she might have said, "Hey, it's so pretty out. Why don't you go take your motorcycle out for a ride?" I just love this! The concept is so simple and yet so *very* effective. The happier the couple, the healthier and happier the environment and the energy in which the children will grow.

"Appreciation can make a day, even change a life.
Your willingness to put it into words is all that is necessary."
—Margaret Cousins

IDENTIFYING STRENGTHS AND WEAKNESSES

A few years ago, a woman interviewed me to be her doula. I asked her how she felt I could best serve her in the birth room. She explained that she wanted me to support, nurture, and coach her, which is part of what a doula does. "How can your husband help you best?" I asked her. She explained, "Just him being there is enough to make me feel safe." She then added, "I love my husband beyond words, and he is amazing at a lot of things, but being nurturing and calming are not his strengths. In fact, that's why I want to hire you."

Smart girl, I thought. This woman knew who this man of hers was, and instead of asking him to be something he wasn't, she hired me to help her in areas out of his comfort zone. How many times do we try to get our partners to show up in ways that they just aren't capable of?

We all have our strengths as well as our limits. I'm not saying you shouldn't ask for what you need—definitely do. It's important to give your partner a chance to come through. But no one person can be everything. And expecting your partner to be everything is totally unrealistic and adds a lot of pressure and responsibility.

Here are some things you can do to have more realistic expectations of your partner and meet both of your needs during and after childbirth.

- **Before the birth, make a list of your partner's strengths.** So often, we point out to our partners what they are doing wrong instead of what they do right. It's best to focus on the positive. What are your partner's strengths? What do you respect and value about him? Where does he shine?

- **With this list, create ways for your partner to be able to help you during birth and after.** By focusing on his strengths and where he shines, he'll be able to easily do what you ask and feel good about helping.

- **Know his (and your) limits.** Like I said above, no one person can give you everything you need. Make a list of your partner's limits and then, using this list, write ways that you can adjust your energy accordingly. For example: One of my clients has a nurturing, loving husband who's a great father but can't clean or cook at all. Instead of asking him to help out in those areas, she hands the baby over to him and has food delivered or has her mother or sister come help. That having been said, give your partner a chance—ask for what you need. If he isn't able to meet your needs, grab your list and put another plan in motion.

- **Be a team player.** Create a list of values, morals, and parenting styles. Even though you're on the same team, not all players on the team have the same jobs. In most relationships, there is a yin/yang energy—one is stronger in certain areas where the other might be weaker. When playing together on a team, this difference completes and strengthens the team as a whole. Both you and your partner should write out the way you hope to parent, including the values and morals you wish to bring into your family, and come up with a game plan.

- **Patch it up.** Go to therapy, talk with each other about your needs, do the above exercises together, and practice accepting who your partner is *now* instead of dwelling on who she isn't or who you wish she would be. People only change when they are ready and want to.

Don't compare partners. Just because your sister's husband may get up every night with their baby, or your best friend's partner changes diapers all the time and yours doesn't, it doesn't mean your partner is at fault. Everyone has different coping skills and operating systems. If you find yourself comparing your partner to others, it is best to bring your focus back to your family and the strengths of the person with whom you chose to have a child.

"We can never obtain peace in the outer world until we make peace with ourselves."

—the 14th Dalai Lama

TANTRIC RELATIONSHIP BONDING MEDITATION

Eye gazing is a great way to connect more deeply with your partner. It allows you to be more present with each other, awakens the heart, and fosters intimacy. Sit facing each other either on the floor or on comfortable chairs. Begin by silently gazing into each other's eyes and holding that gaze for a minute or so. Don't look away, even if you feel uncomfortable at first. Just take in the other person—see them and let them see you. Think and feel in your heart all of the things you appreciate and love about your partner, and let that gratitude and love shine out through your eyes. Hold each other's gaze as long as you can. Afterward, take turns telling each other what you felt about the other.

A CONVERSATION WITH YOUR INNER CHILD

Michele Meiche is a spiritual life coach, healer, and natural psychic who focuses on useful tools for transformation, healing, and empowerment for life enhancement. She created this exercise, which uses guided imagery, visualization, and meditation techniques to help you identify with your inner child and create an open dialogue with him or her to begin a healing process.

To begin, go to a place or create a space that feels safe to you—preferably a place where you won't be disturbed midprocess. Think about your present circumstances. Maybe there's an issue or concern you have. Or you could just be curious. Whatever reason you have for connecting with this hidden part of you is the right reason, one that you don't need to justify to anyone else.

Write in your journal or on a piece of paper:

1. Hello. May I talk with you?
2. I am here to get to know you better.
3. I would like to know more about you.
4. I am now here for you; whether I was a lot or a little in the past, I am more and more fully here for you.
5. What do you need from me at this time?
6. How can we be closer?
7. How can I listen to you better? What does this part of me need to heal?

When you ask these questions and make these statements in your own mind and in your own time, you may or may not get full answers. Sometimes you won't receive anything verbal, just, perhaps, a feeling. Stick with the process consistently. Just like any good relationship or friendship, it takes time to trust one another. There may be some trust issues between you and your inner child. So take the time. You are worth it.

First, get into a comfortable, relaxed position. Close your eyes. Begin focusing on your breath and your heart-lung area. Allow your breath to slow down. Focus on yourself and how you are feeling. Breathe in for a count of 3. Hold for a count of 3. Breathe out for a count of 3. Do this a few times until you feel more relaxed and focused on your inner state. Now, start the conversation with your inner child.

Focus within and, without censoring yourself, note your answers either mentally or by writing them in your journal. (I suggest writing them down.) Do this with each question and take as long as you like. You will know when you're finished when you have a feeling of neutrality, completion, or being more settled.

Feel free to ask as many questions as you'd like. This is your relationship with the inner aspect of yourself. Be respectful and compassionate with the information you receive. You are building trust and learning about a deeper part of you. This all takes time. The more you invest, the better the quality of the relationship and your understanding. Love and accept yourself. This inner part has so much to share with you!

Next-Level Process

After you have developed more rapport with your inner child and feel more trusting, you can begin to have a real partnership with this aspect of yourself.

Ask:

1. What did you need when you were a child that you did not get?

2. How can you get that now in a healthy way? List some ways.

3. How can I (the healthy adult self) provide this?

4. What are you anxious about or afraid of now?

(continued)

Tell your inner child:

1. I am here now—listening, hearing, acknowledging. I understand so much more now about you.

2. You deserve:
   - Unconditional love
   - A safe environment
   - The right to be
   - The right to feel and express your feelings

3. You need to know that:
   - All of your feelings are okay.
   - It's okay to acknowledge them.
   - Feelings are different than actions. You may feel feelings and acknowledge these feelings, yet you may choose to respond or behave differently.
   - It's important to acknowledge and express feelings to your adult self.
   - I am here now and listening to your needs.
   - You have the right to be heard, acknowledged, and understood.
   - I understand why you feel what you feel.
   - You have a right to full self-expression, to create and express yourself.
   - Others may not always agree with how you are feeling or what you think, but you are entitled to have and express your feelings.

So many times we are so much more understanding of other people and so critical of ourselves. Just look at how far you have come in your life. Look at what you've overcome. Look at the challenges and how you've made it through.

Create comfort and safety for your inner child. Release fear and anxiety by listening, hearing, acknowledging, understanding, and honoring this part of you.

"When eye contact between two people is initiated and maintained, an invisible energetic circuit is established between the two participants, dissolving the barriers that ordinarily separate them from each other, drawing them ever closer into a shared awareness of union."

—Will Johnson

HOW TO HANDLE A COLD OR THE FLU

You might find yourself sick at some point during your pregnancy. This isn't unusual, no matter how careful you are about avoiding sick people. Your body is working extra hard just to be pregnant, and it's more susceptible to colds and other illnesses. Here are some simple, natural ways to take care of yourself when you have a cold or flu.

- Steam yourself. Breathing in steam does wonders for your nasal passages and congested chest. You can get the same effect in a few ways. First, hold your head over a pot of boiling water and breathe through your nose. (Be careful, though, as the steam can be a little too hot at first.) A humidifier works the same way but lasts longer than a pot of water on the stove. Finally, turn your shower all the way up and close the bathroom door. Sit on the toilet or near the shower and deeply breathe in the steam that will fill up the room. Stay there as long as you can handle it. For all of these methods, adding five drops of eucalyptus oil to the water (or the shower floor) will further help clear your breathing passages.

- Use nasal strips, a great natural and nonmedicinal way to open up your sinuses. Place one nasal strip over your nose, and it will gently pull your nasal passages open. This helps the most when you're trying to sleep.

- Try this homeopathic remedy: Take one tube of oscillococcinum every 6 hours (three tubes total daily) at the first sign of a cold or flu.

- Use a neti pot with a saline rinse to flush out your sinuses.

- Stay hydrated with water or tea. You can also try my homemade sports drink recipe (8 ounces of coconut water, one Emergen-C packet, and a pinch of Himalayan sea salt).

- Take a damp washcloth and heat it for 30 seconds in a microwave. Place it over your congested sinuses for temporary relief.

- Rest and sleep! The more rest you get, the faster you will heal.

- Drink a combination of ginger and peppermint tea. Ginger is a natural decongestant and peppermint helps control coughs. My favorite way to make this is to put chopped fresh ginger and a few sprigs of mint in a mug and pour hot water over them. Let it steep for a few minutes, and add honey and some lemon!

- Gargle with ½ teaspoon of sea salt mixed with warm water. You can also gargle with or drink 1 teaspoon of apple cider vinegar in warm water. Drinking this mixture helps soothe sore throat symptoms.

- Suck on a zinc throat lozenge.

- Make your own vapor chest rub. Melt ½ cup of coconut oil and ¼ cup of beeswax (you can find beeswax pregrated or in pebble form) and place the mixture in a small glass jar. Mix in 10 drops of eucalyptus oil and 4 drops of peppermint oil. Rub on your chest. Keep this in a sealed container in a cool, dry place.

- Take echinacea, which boosts the immune system to help prevent colds, flu, and infections.

- Eat vitamin C–rich foods such as citrus fruits, berries, sweet potato, melon, and broccoli.

- Take a good probiotic to help strengthen your immune system.

- Avoid dairy products, as they produce extra mucus.

Stefani's Hand-Me-Down Chicken Soup

Chicken soup has been a staple in my coauthor Stefani's family for both holidays and the winter cold and flu season. With so many different women in her family giving her chicken soup recipes through the years, she decided to take the best from each one to create her own style of soup.

1 cut-up organic fryer chicken

1 organic chicken bouillon cube, preferably without MSG

2 parsnips, chopped into large pieces

4 carrots, cut into 2" pieces

2 bay leaves

Handful of flat, whole parsley sprigs

1 onion, quartered

1 package (12 ounces) No Yolks egg noodles

Salt and pepper

Rinse the chicken in cold water and place it in a large stockpot. Cover the chicken completely with water, almost to the top of the pot.

Cook over medium-high heat until the water starts boiling. White, foamy fat will start bubbling to the top of the pot. Skim the fat out of the pot.

When there's very little fat left to skim, add the bouillon cube, parsnips, carrots, bay leaves, parsley, and onion.

Partially cover the pot. Simmer for 3 to 4 hours. (Two hours is okay, but the longer, the better.)

Strain the soup when it's ready, and be sure to reserve the veggies and chicken and discard the bay leaves and parsley.

Meanwhile, cook the noodles according to package directions until they're al dente.

Add the chicken and veggies back into the soup. Add salt and pepper to taste.

Add the noodles just before serving.

PREGNANCY AND CARPAL TUNNEL SYNDROME

With more and more people constantly texting, e-mailing, and using smartphones and computers these days, I've seen a huge increase in carpal tunnel syndrome among my clients. Carpal tunnel syndrome is caused by pressure from fluids or repetitive movements on the median nerve in the wrist. Symptoms are tingling, numbness, and pain in the hands, fingers, and wrists. Carpal tunnel syndrome can occur at any time during pregnancy, but I've seen it start mostly in the third trimester. It goes away shortly after birth.

Here are some natural ways to alleviate carpal tunnel syndrome. (If it's unbearable, ask your caregiver about possible physical therapy options. These usually involve massage or heat or cold therapy, as well as exercises you can do at home.)

- Massage homeopathic Traumeel cream or St. John's wort oil into your wrists in the mornings and evenings.

- Try acupuncture to get energy and circulation moving.

- Put ice on your wrists for 10 minutes. (Ice shrinks inflamed tissue.) Then soak your wrists in hot water with Epsom salts for 10 minutes. Keep alternating.

- Avoid repetitive movements with your hands when possible.

- Take breaks from the computer to avoid overexertion of your wrists.

- Stretch your hands forward and backward to help increase circulation.

- Wear wrist splints, which you can buy at most pharmacies. Sleep with them on while keeping your hands slightly elevated on a pillow.

- Take vitamin B_6 (25 milligrams daily) and a vitamin B complex for 2 weeks. These vitamins help with swelling and nerve support.

- Exercise regularly to keep your circulation moving and help with swelling.

- Try regular massages to keep your circulation moving. Massage your entire arm with lavender and eucalyptus oils.

- Try this stretch: Get on the floor on all fours with your hands palms down, shoulder-width apart, fingers facing toward your knees. Slowly push your butt back toward your heels, and hold.

Mood-Boosting Smoothie

In life, you'll have good days and bad days. Some days you'll need a little extra pick-me-up and a good dose of positive energy! This is a light, healthy drink that also manages to satisfy a sweet tooth or craving. Vanilla almond milk contains protein and cacao (raw chocolate) is rich in antioxidants, iron, and magnesium to help calm the nerves and relax. Chocolate also helps boost mood, fights fatigue, and naturally energizes the body.

About 5 ice cubes

1 large organic banana, sliced

1 cup vanilla almond milk (organic and unsweetened)

2 tablespoons vanilla whey protein powder

1 tablespoon cacao powder

1 tablespoon flaxseed oil

1 tablespoon chia powder

Honey, agave, or stevia to taste

Place the ice cubes in the bottom of a strong blender. Add the banana, almond milk, protein powder, cacao powder, oil, chia powder, and honey, agave, or stevia. Blend on high speed until smooth. For a thinner consistency, add more almond milk.

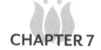

CHAPTER 7

Month Seven

BEING PRESENT

"If you worry about what might be, and wonder what might have been, you will ignore what is."

—Unknown

Welcome to the third and final trimester of your pregnancy! You may still be enjoying the honeymoon phase of pregnancy, when you're not too uncomfortable and hopefully have few physical issues. Now is the perfect time to explore what many of us have a difficult time accomplishing—being truly present with our families, ourselves, and in life in general. These days, we are all multitasking our way through life. Count how many times a day you catch yourself on your cell phone, talking or texting, while eating your lunch or walking down the street. How many times a week do you find yourself thinking, "There just aren't enough hours in the day"? Our ultra-fast-paced lifestyles make us feel like time has sped up and we can't possibly get everything done.

When we multitask, we end up doing a lesser job than if we actually took the time to focus on the task at hand. And by doing three things at once, you can never be *really* fully present or actually engaged in what you're doing. Think how this applies to parenting. We all know how quickly children grow up—consider how fast your pregnancy is going! If we aren't present with our kids, one day we might wonder how we missed so much of their growth. Time is something you can never get back. On the other hand, if you can take the time to be present with yourself, your children, your partner, and your friends, you'll teach your children to do the same by being a living example of what being present and focused looks like.

Being present also means tuning in to the one person who counts on you the most: yourself. While you already wear many hats—wife, partner, daughter, friend—you're about to take on the biggest role of your life. This is a great time to practice being present with yourself, noticing the world around you and how it affects you. This also means being present with uncomfortable feelings and emotions, instead of tuning them out. When you are all right with discomfort and can feel and work through your uncomfortable emotions easily, you will have a better ability to help your children with any difficult emotions they may have.

Obviously, nobody can be 100 percent present all the time. This chapter will help you discover ways to lead by example for your children, to dive in and enjoy what you are doing more fully. After all, it's not how much time you spend with your children that matters but *how* you choose to spend that time. How will you be present today?

YOUR CHANGING BODY

The seventh month of pregnancy is a big turning point for your body. At the start of your third trimester, you're hopefully still feeling pretty comfortable. Month Seven is an ideal time to have pregnancy photos taken, if you want them. Your blood pressure will go up this month, back to what it was before you were pregnant. You might start experiencing shortness of breath. Remind yourself to take slow and deep breaths a few times a day to get more oxygen. Since your belly will really start to grow in Month Seven, you may experience itchy skin. Use Breggy's All-Natural Belly Butter (see page 80) or belly oil a few times a day on your belly, hips, and breasts, if you haven't already started.

Rib pain is common starting in your seventh month. Your uterus is growing in all directions, and rib pain is caused by the uterus pressing into the abdomen and your ribs, as well as baby kicking the area. The pain will likely go away when your baby drops into your pelvic cavity in preparation for birth. Here are a few ways to naturally relieve rib pain.

- Wear loose-fitting clothes. The less pressure you have on your belly and ribs, the easier it is to breathe.
- Support yourself with cushions when sitting or lying down.
- Sit up straight! By not hunching over, you'll create more room in your chest while still supporting your back.
- Avoid sitting down for too long. Take regular stretching breaks or short walks.
- Place heat packs or cold packs under your breasts.
- Float in a pool or warm bath.
- See a chiropractor for an adjustment.
- Try prenatal massage to help relax your body.

A University of Montreal study found that just 20 minutes of moderate exercise, done three times a week, can enhance your baby's brain development.

YOUR GROWING BABY

Your baby is about the size of a butternut squash or head of cabbage, and is an average of 14 inches long. He weighs an average of 2 to 4 pounds. Until this month, your baby's eyes have been sealed shut to protect them and allow the retinas to develop. Now, all the components that make up the eyes are fully developed, allowing the baby's eyelids to begin opening and closing. His eyebrows and lashes have formed, and the hair on his head is now longer. (Of course, you can have a baby with a full head of hair or one who is bald.)

There are some other fabulous things going on with your little one. Your child's hands are now fully developed, complete with tiny nails. Your baby can now curl his hands into fists, and he may even start sucking his thumb. If you have an ultrasound during this time, your baby may be a bit camera shy, covering his face with his curious hands. Your baby will now begin to explore the environment inside your uterus, and you may see a little fist- or heel-size bump appear as he reaches out to feel around his current home. His fingerprints and footprints are now formed as well.

Here's an amazing part of Month Seven: Your baby is able to hear your voice *above* the sound of your heartbeat. I mentioned reading and singing to your baby starting at Month Five. If you've been trying that, wonderful! Now is also a good time to get into the habit of talking, reading, and singing to your baby, since he can actually recognize the sound of your voice. Don't worry if you can't carry a tune. Your baby doesn't care. Sing or hum your favorite songs.

You may be surprised to find your baby calmer and more engaged with you when you read books or sing songs after birth, since your voice is so familiar to her. The more familiar your voice is to your baby, the easier it will be for your voice to soothe the baby after birth. Ask your partner or anyone who is going to be around the baby a significant amount of time to talk or sing along, as well.

BEING PRESENT

"The only true thing is what's in front of you right now."

—Ramona Ausubel

When you live in the present moment, you'll find that the journey is where all the magic happens. The journey is where you find all the lessons and the gifts that each precious moment holds. Sadly, many of us go through life with blinders on, just like a horse racing to the finish line, only seeing the end result. When we live this way, we disconnect from life itself.

Think back on your childhood. What happy memories do you have of times you and your family spent together? Rather than *how much time* you spent with your parents or grandparents, I'm sure it's *how* you were engaged that you remember the most. Perhaps your happiest memories include afternoons at the park, learning to ride a bike, cooking together, or playing cards. Special moments don't need to be fancy occasions, just regular events—but they do need parents or family members to be present and engaged.

When new moms have anxiety about having to go back to work or leaving their child for the first time, I always assure them by saying, "It's not how much time you spend with your children that matters but the way you choose to spend that time with them that does." I remind them that being a living example of what they are trying to teach can be the best form of guidance.

That's why it's so important to practice being mindful in the present moment. We can often feel overwhelmed by the amount of responsibility and pressure normal life holds. When we aren't grounded, we become disconnected and unable to focus on what's right in front of us in this very moment. After all, the past is gone and the future hasn't happened yet—this beautiful moment in time is all we really have. Each choice you make, how you act in the present moment, is a stepping-stone toward building your baby's and your family's future.

USE YOUR SENSES

"Lose your mind and come to your senses."

—Frederick Perl

Our five senses—taste, hearing, sight, smell, and touch—help us to explore and enjoy the world around us. Here are some ways you can play around with each of your senses, to help connect you more to the here and now.

Taste

As a mom-to-be growing a little person, you know that food isn't merely for sustenance. From the moment you learned that you were pregnant, you may have realized that food is one of the only things about your pregnancy that you can control. With every meal, you're choosing exactly which nutrients your baby receives, developing both her body and brain, as well as nourishing your own body.

While you're eating, practice focusing on your food. Take in the colors of the foods on your plate. Bring your attention to the way you chew your foods, and notice how fast and how many times you chew before you swallow. Are you shoveling your meal into your mouth, or do you eat slowly and take a breath or two before your next bite? Feel the food in your mouth and notice the texture; is it smooth, soft, hard, or spongy? Notice the flavors: Does the food taste salty, sour, sweet, or spicy? Feel how grateful you are for this food and how it is feeding and nourishing both you and your baby.

Did you know that your baby will monitor your tone of voice and react to it, too? For example, if you smile at him while talking in a frightened voice, he will still become agitated.

Hearing

Listening to the sounds in your environment is one of the best ways I have found to ground yourself in the here and now. Listen to birds chirp, people talking, and cars going by. Notice how these noises affect you. Do they calm you, aggravate you, or make you happy? Play some music and listen to the beat, the words, the sounds and rhythms that each instrument makes. Notice how different music makes you feel.

Just as you focused on the music, focus and listen when your spouse or a friend is talking to you. Pay attention to what he is saying without intending to answer, but just to hear his opinion or statement. Everyone wants to be heard, and people will tell you all you need to know if you simply drop in and listen.

Sight

Open your eyes—really *open* them! Take in the beauty of life around you; notice the colors, shapes, and textures that surround you. Watch the people you pass and notice how each one is unique. When speaking with someone, show respect by making eye contact. Something you can try on your daily drive or walk home is to stay off the phone and really focus on the road and on noticing your surroundings. If you start daydreaming, bring your mind back to your drive or walk. You will be amazed at all you have missed seeing up until now.

Smell

Many pregnant women have a very heightened sense of smell, so pregnancy is an especially good time for this exercise. Notice the smells wherever you go, noticing both what appeals to you and what doesn't. Smell what you're eating before you taste it, to appreciate your food. Take the time to smell the flowers, the laundry, and the air outside. Do certain smells trigger memories of past events or people?

Using your sense of smell can also help calm you down. Lavender oil is wonderful for its calming properties. Try this easy remedy that you can use every day: Put a few drops of lavender oil on a cotton ball. Carry it around with you, in your pocket or under your bra strap, or put it inside your pillow, and smell it frequently. Lavender is a wonderful scent to help relax and flush your senses. Remember to use oil sparingly—three or four drops per cotton ball will be enough to last for hours.

Your baby's sense of smell is much stronger than yours. She will use it to get to know you in the early weeks after birth. Try to avoid strong perfumes, deodorants, or soaps, and be aware that some household smells may be quite overpowering for her.

Touch

Touch and texture are going to be very important for your newborn because your baby's skin will be supersensitive. Think about everything you will dress or cover your baby in, or how the water temperature needs to be perfectly warm so your baby isn't too hot or cold when taking a bath. Look at your world through a newborn's eyes—you may be surprised at how everything feels.

Feel the different textures and surfaces all around you. If you have a pet, notice how its fur feels. When you hug someone, feel her body against yours and see if you can feel her energy. Touch someone and feel his skin—is it hot or cold, dry or moist? When eating, feel the food in your mouth and notice the texture. Walk barefoot and feel the earth supporting you. Feel the sun's heat on you or the wind blowing on your body. When you shower, feel the water on your body and notice the temperature; what feels better, hot or cold?

"When we are willing to stay even a moment with uncomfortable energy, we gradually learn not to fear it."
—Pema Chödrön

Touch is one of your baby's most advanced senses at birth. Even premature babies born as early as 25 weeks are aware of being touched. Your baby's sense of touch develops from head to toe, and the mouth is the first region to become sensitive. This is why young babies put *everything* in their mouths.

BEING PRESENT WITH YOURSELF

If we can't be alone, present, and okay with ourselves—the good, the bad, *and* the ugly—how will we have the ability to be present and okay with all aspects of our children?

I used to teach a weekly yoga class and would ask my students to hold deep stretches for long periods of time. I had them breathe into the stretch and feel the tightness in their muscles and joints. After a few rounds of this breathing, I had them name the sensation they felt. Some people would name it "pain," "stress," "protection," or "tension." I asked them to stay with their named sensation, breathing in healing energy through the "in" breath and exhaling out any discomfort.

As students did this exercise, their bodies would let go and open up as they began to go deeper into their stretches. After a while, I had them ask themselves, "What am I holding in here? What emotion or feeling is under this sensation?" Some people felt frustration, anger, sadness, or loneliness. Again I had them sit, feel, and breathe into that feeling. This is when most of the class usually started to fidget, look around, zone out, or take themselves out of the pose.

How often in life do we do the same thing? We start to feel too much emotion; the feeling gets uncomfortable, so we take ourselves out of it. We distract ourselves, staying as busy as we can so we don't have to experience uncomfortable feelings. Finally, we shut down, close off, or numb ourselves with food, work, or other distractions to avoid discomfort at all costs.

The last thing I asked my students to do in this exercise was to explore that feeling or emotion that they were carrying. I had them think about how it manifested itself in their lives and where it came from. I had them breathe in the opposite of the feeling—if they felt sadness, I had them breathe *in* happiness and exhale *out* the sadness in their life. After just sitting and being with these feelings for a while, amazing things began to happen. People's energy shifted from pain and suffering to a sense of relaxation and peace.

We can only sweep things under the rug for so long before they start to pile up and spill out again. When we are able to sit with and feel our pain, explore it and process it, the energy begins to dissipate. You don't need to be in a yoga pose to be present with yourself and work through your "stuff." You just need to make time by allowing yourself to be alone, drop in, and feel. When we aren't able to be there for ourselves and understand our own pain and suffering, how can we be there for another? As a mother, there will be days when your child is sad, angry, or just having a hard day. The more you can be there for yourself, feeling comfortable with and acknowledging your own emotions, the more you can empathize and feel compassion for other people's feelings and emotions.

"The future is completely open, and we are writing it moment to moment."

—Pema Chödrön

NATURAL REMEDIES FOR VARICOSE VEINS

Varicose veins are bluish, bulging veins that appear on your legs at the surface of your skin. While varicose veins are generally not painful, they can be uncomfortable. The exact cause of varicose veins is not known, but a genetic tendency toward weak vein valves plays a role.

Hormones also play a big part in varicose veins, so pregnant women are very prone to developing them. During pregnancy, the increased blood volume you're circulating for yourself and your baby can make veins bulge. Sitting with a full uterus on the top of your thighs also prevents blood from returning to the heart effectively. Many varicose veins that pop up during pregnancy deflate in 3 months, although new pregnancies can bring them on again, sometimes to stay.

The bad news is that varicose veins are sometimes unavoidable. The good news? There are many ways to naturally prevent and soothe them. Here are a few suggestions.

- Get plenty of exercise to get your blood circulating.

- Elevate your legs daily on pillows for 10 minutes or more.

- Avoid excess weight gain.

- Dry-brush your legs daily to improve circulation. (This can prevent varicose veins from forming.) Use a natural bristle brush with a long handle, so you can reach all parts of your body. Gently brush your legs from the ankles up in a circular motion. Do this before you shower, so you can wash off any dead skin you brush off. Follow with moisturizer or body oil to achieve super soft and glowing skin! However, don't do this on any existing varicose veins because you may irritate them.

- Take sociable garlic and vitamin E capsules to improve circulation and vitamin C and B-complex vitamins to strengthen your blood vessels.

- Massage your legs with upward strokes, flushing your blood up to your heart. Use three drops of lavender oil with one drop of peppermint oil in a coconut oil base (use unscented coconut oil), or put only the essential oils into a small spray bottle filled with water and spray directly on your legs.

St. John's wort oil also helps with inflammation of veins. You can buy or make the oil yourself with just a couple of ingredients. Place a few handfuls of the plant (I use the dried flowers) in a Mason jar. Fill the rest of the jar with cold-pressed, organic olive oil (leave a little space at the top). Store in a cool, dry place and it will stay fresh for a month.

- Avoid sitting too long, especially with your legs crossed.
- Wear loose clothing.
- Try acupuncture or reflexology treatments to get your circulation moving and to move any stagnant energy.
- After a bath, apply castor oil directly onto the veins. Massage using upward strokes from your feet straight up your legs.
- Avoid standing for prolonged periods of time.
- Apply a cool compress soaked in witch hazel on your legs. Add a few drops of rosemary oil to stimulate circulation.
- Flex your feet up and down and circle your ankles to the left and to the right twice a day.
- Try wearing compression stockings or support pantyhose.

To help varicose veins, make sure you're getting enough of the following:

- Calcium-rich foods, since varicose veins are aggravated by a calcium deficiency
- Pineapple, to reduce swelling and inflammation
- Berries such as raspberries, blackberries, blueberries, and cherries, as they contain a pigment that strengthens the walls of the veins
- Foods high in fiber
- Plenty of water, to keep your bowels moving

> "Look deep into nature and then you will understand everything better."
> —Albert Einstein

WALKING MEDITATION

Walking is a great exercise that almost anyone can do daily during pregnancy. Here's a simple walking meditation to bring presence of mind and body; you can practice it each time you step outside for a stroll. Begin simply by paying attention to your feet; watch them, feel the ground underneath them, and listen to the sound of them hitting the ground as you walk. Notice the sounds in the air—birds chirping or leaves on the trees moving in the wind. If there's a river or stream nearby, listen to its rhythm. If your mind starts wandering, bring your attention back to your feet and the sounds, smells, and sights all around you. Take in the smells of the flowers and the cut grass. Open your eyes and view the different colors and textures around you, such as the leafy green trees and bright yellow flowers, brown squirrels, fluffy white clouds, and deep blue sky. Feel the sun heating up your body and the air surrounding you. If you are walking a dog, listen to its breathing and footsteps as well. There are so many sensations happening all around you at all times.

If your mind starts to wander at any time, label it as "thinking," and then bring your attention back to your surroundings. If you see a bird, bug, or animal, watch it for a while. If you start daydreaming or worrying, again label it as "thinking," and bring your attention back to your walk and the here and now. Doing this often helps train your mind to be focused and present in the moment and helps you become aware of your thinking mind. It also helps you to notice the beauty around you that otherwise might be overlooked when you're distracted.

"Children are natural Zen masters;
their world is brand new in each and every moment."
—John Bradshaw

CLEARING YOUR MIND

Overthinking prevents us from being here in the now. How often do you find yourself awake at night, stressing out about something—whether it's bigger issues like what your labor will be like or your finances or little things like whether you remembered to return that baby gift you don't really need? Too often, your mind will worry about things that, at three o'clock in the morning, you can do little about. Do the following breathing meditation for just a few minutes a day and try to work up to 20 minutes a day. Set a timer if that helps allow you to truly clear your head for this brief exercise.

Sit in a cross-legged position with your eyes closed. Begin to focus on your breath, and start to inhale through your nose slowly for a count of 4. Take deep breaths into your belly and baby. Then exhale through your nose for 4 slow counts. Keep repeating— 4 counts breathing in through your nose and 4 counts breathing out through your nose.

When you perform this basic meditation, try to recognize your wandering mind every time little thoughts take you away from breathing, label it as "thinking," and then bring your focus back to your breath. Be a witness to your mind and the voice in your head. You can tune it out just by bringing the focus back to your breathing, as meditation is what you're doing *in the moment*. The more often you do this meditation, the easier it will be. After your mind is calm, you will hear another voice from deep within you—the voice of your inner guidance. You can't hear that voice with an active mind.

WRITING EXERCISE: BE PRESENT WITH YOUR PARTNER

How are you and your partner present for each other? How do you show love for each other beyond the typical gestures or physical contact? Of course, being intimate with your partner is an important aspect of being there for one another. But there are many other ways you can let your partner know you love, appreciate, and respect who she is and how important her support is to you. Doing this mindfully allows you to be present in your relationship, instead of letting the days and your actions slip by without a thought.

Make a list of ways you and your partner show love and appreciation for one another. Do you have a monthly date night at a special restaurant? Leave notes by the bedside each morning?

Maybe you enjoy listening to music together while you have dinner, or you plan and cook one meal together each week. Or maybe you simply say "I love you" before you each go to work. If you've begun doing these things thoughtlessly—or not at all—maybe now's a good time to remind yourself that these moments or actions, however small, help keep your relationship strong. Affection doesn't have to be limited to gifts or date nights. Children will see you and your partner interact on many levels, even when you think they aren't paying attention.

BRINGING YOUR ENERGY TO THE PRESENT

When life gets crazy, remember to bring yourself back to the present moment to find calmness and a whole new perspective. I practice the technique below to bring my own energy back into the present moment before I see a client, to make sure I'm in the space I need to be to pay attention to the woman I'll be working with. My work is intuitive and instinctual, and I need to be in the moment and give my full attention to all of my clients. Try it!

- Plant your feet firmly on the ground or sit comfortably in a chair.
- Feel the ground or the chair beneath you.
- Say your full name, today's date, and the time.
- Look at yourself and mentally notice your clothes and your appearance. Scan your body, name different aspects of your appearance, and begin to label them. For example, "I'm wearing black sneakers, a cream-colored sweater, blue jeans; I have red nails; my hair is in a bun; I have blue eyes," etc.
- Take notice of your surroundings and label them. For example, "I'm in my home, in my living room; there's a wood coffee table in front of me; candles are burning; my dog is next to me on the off-white couch," etc.

🍃 Take a deep breath and breathe in the present moment. Next, exhale it out.

Remember, the only thing you have control over is this moment. The past is gone and the future hasn't happened yet. What you do in the here and now sets the tone for everything beyond today, for you, your baby, and your family.

QUICK FOOT MASSAGE

This is a great exercise for both grounding yourself *and* massaging your sore feet. A simple tennis ball is all you need. It's inexpensive and you can do it at home, at the office, or while traveling, whenever you want.

Here's how it works.

1. Start by placing the tennis ball in the center of your foot by your arch. Take a deep breath and, as you exhale, put your weight on the ball and allow your foot to slowly melt around the ball like butter melting in the hot sun. Gently hold your foot there until the tension subsides.

2. Close your eyes and slowly roll the ball around your foot, exploring your foot for sore spots. When you find a tight area, again slowly take a deep breath and, as you exhale, put your weight on the ball and feel the knotted area. Release your foot as you exhale. Keep doing this until all the tightness in your foot is gone.

3. Repeat with the other foot.

4. When you're finished, stand with both feet on the floor. Bring attention to your feet and feel how much more grounded to the earth you are.

Yoga for Rib Pain

Gentle yoga stretches can also help with sore ribs. Try these on a daily basis, and find one or two poses that work for you.

SUPPORTED SIDE STRETCH

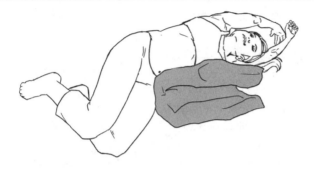

Start by kneeling. Sit your butt down toward your heels, then slide it to the left and to the floor. Place a rolled-up towel or bolster alongside your left hip. Walk your left hand and arm all the way down so you're lying sideways over the bolster. Move your rib cage backward slightly. Now, place your right arm over your head. Inhale deep into your ribs. When you exhale, concentrate on softening your rib cage and chest area.

CHILD'S POSE STRETCH

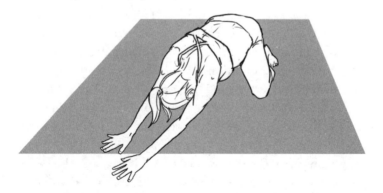

Start in Child's Pose with your arms out in front of you, palms flat on the floor. Begin to crawl both hands over to the left, taking a deep breath into the right side of the rib cage. As you exhale, relax the area.

On the next breath, walk your arms farther to the left and, again, exhale and soften. Do this one more time. Then walk your arms over to the right and repeat. Do three rounds of breaths.

GENTLE TWIST

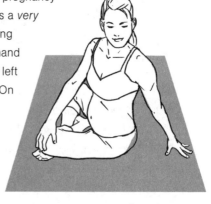

Twists are generally a no-no for pregnancy yoga—except for this one. This is a *very* gentle twist that *is* allowed. Sitting cross-legged, place your right hand on your left knee and walk your left hand a few inches behind you. On each inhale, get a little more length in your spine. When you exhale, go into the twist a little deeper. Repeat the twist on the other side.

EAT SMART

In Month Seven, your baby is experiencing full-on brain development. It's time to focus on eating brain food. The following foods contain omega-3 fatty acids and healthy fats. Taking in enough omega-3s will improve your baby's eye and brain growth and early development and may lower your baby's chances of getting asthma and other allergic conditions, according to a study cited in an abstract published by the NYU Langone Medical Center. Omega-3s can also lower blood pressure, reduce your risk of heart disease and other health problems, and may lower your risk of giving birth too early or of experiencing postpartum depression.

By eating good fats and essential fatty oils, you will also be helping along the accumulation of fat under baby's skin. It's in the seventh month that your child will start gaining weight faster, in part because of this fat layer. Foods that contain these good fats include:

- **Healthy oils:** fish oil, coconut oil, olive oil, canola oil, and flaxseed oil

- **Seeds:** hemp seeds, flaxseeds, sesame seeds, pumpkin seeds, and sunflower seeds
- **Nuts and nut butters:** walnuts, pecans, almonds
- **Beans and legumes:** soybeans and lentils
- **Leafy green veggies:** spinach, kale, collard greens, and cabbage
- **Vegetables** such as avocado, squash, and cauliflower
- **Fish** such as cod, salmon, and anchovies

Roasted Root Veggies

Root vegetables are great to eat to help ground your energy when life might have you spinning. This is an easy recipe that you can play around with, adding veggies that you love and enjoy and eliminating those you don't. It makes a lot of food but reheats well, so you can serve it with a couple of meals.

2½ pounds butternut squash, peeled, seeded, cut into ½" pieces

1½ pounds Yukon Gold potatoes, unpeeled, cut into ½" pieces

1 yam, unpeeled, cut into ½" pieces

1 bunch beets (about 1½ pounds), trimmed but not peeled, scrubbed, cut into ½" pieces

1 medium red onion, cut into ½" pieces

1 large turnip, peeled, cut into ½" pieces

1 bulb garlic, cloves separated and peeled

2 tablespoons olive oil

Salt, pepper, paprika, rosemary, and thyme to taste

Preheat the oven to 425°F. Oil 2 large rimmed baking sheets. In a large bowl, combine the squash, potatoes, yam, beets, onion, turnip, garlic, and oil. Toss to coat. Spread the veggies in a single layer on the baking sheets and sprinkle generously with the salt, pepper, paprika, rosemary, and thyme. Roast the vegetables until they're tender and golden brown, about 1 hour 15 minutes, stirring occasionally. (To reheat, roast at 350°F for 15 minutes.)

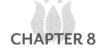

CHAPTER 8

Month Eight

MAKING SPACE FOR BABY

"The secret of change is to focus all of your energy,
not on fighting the old, but on building the new."

—Socrates

Your baby will be here in 8 weeks or less! It's a great time to let go of the old and make room for the new. By now, your nesting instincts have probably kicked in and you may feel an overwhelming need to clean up or get rid of unneeded stuff. This is totally normal and a great way to prepare for your baby. This is the time to let go of the things that you've outgrown or that aren't working, to make room for this next chapter of your life to begin. De-cluttering, both literally and figuratively, means you won't have unnecessary "junk" piling up and taking up space. Just like your physical space, you'll also take inventory of friendships, relationships, and situations in your life that you have outgrown or that no longer serve you, and create some healthy space within them.

I've noticed a pattern with my clients toward the end of their pregnancies: They go through a "nesting period" where they have an uncontrollable urge to purge, clean, and organize their homes and their lives. This can happen at any point during pregnancy, but it's when the due date is getting close that women really begin to feel that instinct to prepare for the new arrival. People nest in all kinds of ways. Some women deep-clean and purge their homes of things such as old clothing, books, and other "stuff." Some have to organize every closet and cabinet. Some feel the need to restructure and rebalance their lives or to pull away from certain people or activities. Others are strictly focused on organizing the nursery and baby clothes.

I once found one of my clients (then 8 months pregnant) in her basement, throwing away boxes of stuff, reorganizing shelves, and scrubbing them clean. When she saw me, she burst into tears. "I can't stop cleaning!" she cried. I explained that this is totally normal. A celebrity client of mine fired her entire staff during her pregnancy. She hired more like-minded people who were a better fit for this new chapter in her life. During pregnancy, there is a natural excitement, anticipation, and nervousness. The nesting urge gives this energy a place to go.

"You can't reach for anything new if your hands are full of yesterday's junk."
—Unknown

When I prepare someone during pregnancy, one of the things I do is to help her create some space in her life by clearing out, letting go, and rearranging. As humans, we're constantly growing and evolving. Having a child is a major life change. Not only will you birth this child, but another part of yourself—a mother—is being born, as well. Nesting is a great way to reevaluate and take inventory of your life. Here are some tips to begin clearing your clutter, both inside and out.

- **Take inventory of your life.** Notice what's working, what needs adjusting, and what needs to go. Look at the way you've been living—we can't change anything if we aren't aware of what needs changing. What can you let go of to make space for the new? When you get rid of what is taking up space—literally and figuratively—you'll have much more breathing room and space for the new to come in.

- **Detox your kitchen and feed your body and mind.** It's always worth the time and energy to scrub your kitchen with the nontoxic cleaners I suggested in Chapter 1. The next step to get your kitchen ready is to stock it full of the foods you've been enjoying throughout your pregnancy. Now that you're thinking more about your baby's arrival, you can get your kitchen ready with foods you'll need right before the birth and postpregnancy. It's never too late to be organized, especially when you'll be a lot busier in a few weeks.

- **Distance yourself from the negative.** Take inventory of your friendships: Who "feeds" you? Who inspires you? Who do you feel good being around? I have different levels of friendships that change as I change. Imagine an archery target. I'm the bull's-eye and my inner circle of friends is that first ring around the bull's-eye. Other relationships fill the rings that go farther out. Ask yourself: Who drains you, who isn't supportive, who are you not on the same wavelength with at the moment? You don't want people around the bull's-eye crowding out the folks who you resonate with. Figure out who needs to be moved to the outer rings. That doesn't mean they can't come back in at a later time. This allows for flexibility and space with relationships without cutting people completely out of your life.

- **Clean house.** Take the time to look through your house and figure out what can use a good cleaning and purging. That may include going through clothes you and your partner don't wear anymore, food and kitchen supplies that have been lurking in the backs of your cabinets, old makeup and personal supplies, or whatever else is taking up unwanted space in your home. Throw away old papers, give old books to your local library, or hold a garage sale. I guarantee you'll feel like you have more room to breathe while you're getting your home ready for baby.

- **Patch the energy leaks.** You're about to embark on the most amazing journey of your life. Becoming a parent allows you to reevaluate what's important for you and your family. Notice where (or with whom) you are spending too much time, money, or energy, and which may leave you feeling drained. Where can you create more structure and establish better boundaries? Patch up the leaks that are draining your energy away so you have more of it for the important things in life.

What about people you're close with—how can you distance yourself from their negativity? These might be family members or work colleagues you have to be around often. Don't be afraid to limit the time you spend with them and set healthy boundaries. Something happens during pregnancy—you just won't be able to tolerate negativity. It's that protective mama bear coming out! I've mentioned this before, but I can't stress it enough: You can't control others' actions, but you can always control your reactions and how much time and energy you spend with and give to them.

- **Find balance.** We've been talking a lot about finding balance in your life. Later in this chapter, I'll ask you to evaluate aspects of your life that may be throwing you off balance. Are you moving your body enough or taking enough time for yourself? Are you working too much and not finding time to relax? Where can you make changes so you can have a better-balanced life?

YOUR CHANGING BODY

The eighth month of pregnancy is when many women start to feel that true excitement (and nervous anticipation) of knowing their baby will arrive in just 2 short months or less. This month, you might find that many daily activities, like sleeping and breathing, are becoming uncomfortable. Consistent daily walks will help keep your mood and energy up and all of your internal organs functioning smoothly.

Here are some ways you can still get some exercise that won't wear you out.

- Take walks in nature. If that's not an option, use a treadmill or walk somewhere indoors, like your local mall.

- Prenatal yoga is a great source of gentle stretching and breathing practices that will keep you mindful of your body and baby. You may not be able to do everything you could in your early months of pregnancy, so focus on simple, comfortable poses to keep your blood flowing and your limbs loose.

- Swimming is an amazing all-over body exercise that doesn't put a strain on any part of your body. The water will also help you feel lighter and take excess stress off your legs and feet.

- If it's cold outside, consider using a stationary bike or elliptical machine at your local gym, or lift some light weights.

Your breasts might feel very full now. This month, you might see the appearance of colostrum, also called "first milk." It's yellow to orange in color (resembling melted butter) and it's thick

Many women think their baby isn't getting enough milk in the first few days. Did you know that, at Day One, a newborn's stomach is only the size of a cherry and can only hold around 1½ tablespoons of milk? By Day Three, the stomach has grown to the size of a walnut; by the end of Week One, the size of an apricot; and by the end of Month One, about the size of a large egg. It can then hold up to 5 ounces of milk.

and sticky (like maple syrup). It has higher concentrations of sodium, potassium, protein, fat-soluble vitamins, and minerals than mature milk.

Colostrum will be the first milk your baby ingests when breast-feeding. It's a misconception that colostrum isn't enough milk to support your baby during its first couple of days; colostrum contains a gold mine of nutrients to keep your baby satisfied and healthy.

I described Braxton Hicks contractions in Chapter 6 as your uterus practicing for the big day. They may come more frequently now, but they are perfectly harmless (and kind of exciting!). Of course, if you're worried that what you're experiencing is more than Braxton Hicks, call your caregiver. Something I have my clients start doing this month is perineal massage. Perineal massage involves gently kneading the perineum (the delicate area located between the anus and the vagina). Prepping the perineum for childbirth can help prevent or lessen tears or the need for an episiotomy during childbirth. Here's what to do.

- Sit in bed or prop yourself on the floor with a lot of pillows. Bend your knees and get into a position where you won't strain your neck during the massage.

- Make sure your nails are cut short and your hands are clean! You don't want to nick yourself or introduce germs to the perineum.

- Use coconut oil to lubricate your fingers and perineal area.

- Place your thumbs 1 inch inside your vagina. Place the rest of your fingers down by your butt.

- Apply slight pressure down (toward your anus) and out (toward the vaginal walls). Hold here for around 10 seconds or until you feel a stretching sensation. Then, keeping your thumbs pressed down, massage the area in a U-shaped motion for 5 to 10 minutes.

- As the next few weeks go by, you may want to teach your partner how to do perineal massage. It will probably seem awkward at first, but you may not be able to comfortably reach your vagina at the very end of your pregnancy. Consistent massage will be extremely beneficial for you. If you aren't comfortable asking your partner to do this, here's a trick you can try to continue doing it yourself: Sit in the bathtub with your feet on the wall. This position helps to get a good angle for perineal massage.

YOUR GROWING BABY

This month, your baby is going to gain weight faster than ever—she is set to gain more than half her birth weight in these last few weeks alone. By the end of the eighth month, the average weight for a baby is 4½ to 5½ pounds and the average length is 17 to 18 inches. Picture your baby weighing about the same as a large honeydew melon and resembling a long leaf of romaine lettuce.

Your baby still has some wiggle room in there, but at this point you won't be able to ignore every kick, elbow, and roll over as your baby becomes more active. If you lie down on your back, you'll probably be able to see a wave of feet and elbows slowly move across your belly. If you haven't started counting your baby's movements already, your caregiver may tell you to start. By the eighth month, you should be able to feel roughly 10 movements every 2 hours. Of course, this depends on your activity level during the hour you decide to count kicks. At this point, babies have more of an asleep/awake routine (at least, until they're outside the womb). Here are some ways to gently rouse your baby so you can be sure she is still fumbling around inside.

Brain scans have shown evidence that babies have periods of REM (rapid eye movement) sleep, when dreaming occurs, from the eighth month of pregnancy onward.

- Lie down in a quiet place. When your body ceases to move, your baby may wake up and start moving.
- Eat a small snack, such as a piece of fruit. The natural sugars will awaken the baby and make her more active.
- Play music. Your baby may have a musical preference, but I recommend soothing music to comfort her. Try playing classical music or chanting. Once she hears the beat, she may start moving along to it.
- Drink something cold. The temperature change might nudge baby into moving.
- Gently push a couple of fingers into your belly.

If you could touch your baby right now, she would still be covered in lanugo, the downy hair that helps protect skin. By Month Eight, however, that lanugo begins to disappear. Lung development is also extremely important during these final 8 weeks of pregnancy. A fetus's lungs get stronger and stronger as the days progress, so the longer she stays in utero, the better for her lungs.

CREATE YOUR OWN SACRED SPACE IN YOUR HOME

"Your sacred space is where you can find yourself again and again."
—Joseph Campbell

I am a huge fan of creating a sacred space in the home. It can be wherever you want (or have room). If you have the luxury of taking over a whole room, then go for it. If not, it can be a comfortable chair in the corner or a room, a patio, or anywhere else you can find to sit comfortably. My sacred space is in my bedroom. One of my clients even has her sacred space in her bathroom.

Your sacred space is a place where you can recharge, reflect, ground or calm yourself, and replenish. When taking a client through my program, I usually work with her to create a place in her home early in the pregnancy, so she's used to going there by the time the baby arrives. Her space is instilled in her by then as her calm spot, and she will use it as much as she needs.

Your sacred space can be as large or small as you like. One of my clients has a beautiful garden with lots of roses and a fountain. We created her sacred space in it, complete with wind chimes and a hammock hung between two trees, in the shade. The hammock is her sacred space. She goes out there, closes her eyes, and rocks in the hammock, listening to the birds, wind chimes, and fountain. This is her calm spot, her place for peace and reflection. She started using her sacred space early in her pregnancy, and after she gave birth she found that she craved being there. So she brought the baby monitor out back and, when her baby napped, she curled up in her sacred space for a rest as well.

I also have a friend who lives in a small New York City apartment. Even though her space is more limited, she created a wonderful place just for herself. She has a meditation pillow in a corner of a room with a small altar in front of it where she has photos, crystals, flowers, and things that inspire her. She puts on headphones and listens to nature sounds like a flowing river or ocean waves while reflecting, journaling, or meditating.

Fill your sacred space with things that inspire, calm, and replenish your being. Some things that might help to create your sacred space are:

- Flowers or plants
- Candles, incense, essential oils for aromatherapy, and crystals
- Religious symbols
- Positive affirmations or quotes
- Photos of loved ones or vision boards
- Soft lighting
- Books and music
- Comfortable blankets or pillows

By 35 weeks, most babies have settled into the position they'll be in at birth. Many babies will begin to settle into a head-down position in the uterus. This is because the top part of the uterus is larger and allows more room for the biggest part of the baby, which is baby's bottom and bent-up legs.

Remember, this space is for you. Make it a place where you can reflect, read, journal, drink tea, write, nap, draw, meditate—anything you love to do to unwind. The energy of your surroundings holds a space for the way you want to feel. By carving out a space tailored for you—no matter how big or small—you'll always have a place to retreat to when you need it.

CREATING A SACRED SPACE IN THE HOSPITAL

By now, you've probably already decided where you're giving birth. In the back of the book, I've created birth plans for two of the most popular locations: hospital and home. Home births can be a wonderful experience, but not everyone feels comfortable giving birth at home. I try to help all my clients to be well prepared and have a peaceful and positive birth experience, no matter where they physically have their baby.

The typical hospital room can be a pretty sterile environment. There are things you can do, however, to transform the whole vibe of your hospital room. It's important that you feel good in your birth space! When I go into the birth room with a client, the first thing I do is create a sacred space of peace and calm; this space holds the energy for everyone in the room.

Here are a few things you can do to make any birth space (whether at the hospital or in your home) more peaceful.

- **Soften the lights.** Turn off the lights and use the natural daylight. If it's nighttime, light up the room with flameless candles (you can find them on Amazon.com) or bring in a couple of small lamps that give off cozy lighting. One of my clients hung Christmas lights over the windowsill, which definitely made the room more cheerful.

- **Make a playlist.** When preparing my clients for birth, I have them make a birthing playlist of songs that have meaning, that they love, or that they find calming for the baby to enter the world, too. I've found playing healing, spa-like music or chants during labor to be really helpful.

- **Make an altar.** Just like at home, bring to your hospital the altar things that inspire you, calm you, and give you strength. People have brought photos of loved ones (both living and deceased), the baby's ultrasound picture, photos of their dogs, a stuffed animal, or a piece of clothing for the baby. Other ideas: crystals, affirmations, pictures of deities or goddesses, or a picture of your guru. Bring whatever inspires you or whoever's energy you want there with you.

- **Use an aromatherapy diffuser with essential oils.** Bring an electrical aromatherapy diffuser and burn oils throughout the whole birthing process. I massage my clients' heads with sandalwood oil to calm their minds and massage their feet with oils of pine or cedar to help ground their energy. (I'll go into which essential oils I use throughout the labor and delivery experience in the next chapter.)

- **Bring your own pillow and cozy blanket.** I'll talk about this more when I go into packing for the hospital, but bringing these familiar items from home will make you feel super cozy.

- **Be picky about who you allow in the room.** I spoke about this in Chapter 2, when I discussed setting boundaries. Everyone holds certain energies, and this isn't the time to add a stressful person into your sacred and calm space. Only allow into the room the people around whom you feel totally supported. I was once at a birth where the husband's family kept trying to come into the room against his wife's wishes. A nurse said to the husband, "This moment is your rite of passage into fatherhood. It's up to you to protect your wife and baby." She sent him out of the room to deal with his family and uphold his wife's wishes for an undisturbed birth, free of family drama.

MEDITATION: BREATHING LIFE INTO YOUR BABY

Sit in a comfortable position with your eyes closed. Place your hands on each side of your rib cage. Through your nose, slowly take a deep breath into your lungs, filling them all the way up to the top. Hold for 2 or 3 seconds. As you exhale through your nose, allow all the air to come out of the bottom of your ribs and your diaphragm area to soften and relax. Do this three times.

Next, keep doing the same breath, but this time imagine as you fill up your lungs with oxygen that you're also breathing into your baby's lungs, sending him life force energy. Imagine not only your lungs expanding with each breath, but your baby's lungs also expanding and getting stronger. With every breath you take, feed your baby-to-be by breathing life into him. Breathe in life and vitality and exhale, as both your and your baby's lungs become supple and relaxed.

NATURAL RELIEF FOR HEMORRHOIDS

Hemorrhoids in pregnancy are most common during the third trimester. Hemorrhoids are swollen blood vessels in the rectal area that develop from the pressure of your growing uterus and increased bloodflow. They can be itchy and painful and can sometimes cause rectal bleeding, but they will usually go away shortly after the birth of your baby. Try these ways to get natural relief.

- Use chilled witch hazel pads with added vitamin E oil. Witch hazel is a natural astringent and helps heals the swelling and inflammation when applied externally. Pharmacies sell wipes premoistened with witch hazel; however, you can make your own witch hazel pads at home. You can also apply witch hazel directly to the anus using a cotton pad.

- Try taking a sitz bath. The shallow bath cleanses the perineum (the space between the rectum and the vulva). Pharmacies also sell plastic sitz bath kits that will fit over your toilet. I recommend adding ¼ cup of witch hazel and ½ cup of Himalayan or Celtic sea salt, plus three drops of lavender oil, to a shallow tub of warm water. Soak in the sitz bath up to two times per day, for 20 minutes total per day.

- Try using a "donut" pillow whenever you need to sit down, to take pressure off your hemorrhoids.

- Try to avoid constipation, which causes you to strain when using the bathroom, aggravating your existing hemorrhoids or creating more. Keep eating fruits, vegetables, and whole grains, and add fiber to your diet when you can to keep your bowels moving. Drinking prune juice with flaxseeds will also keep your digestive system regular.

- Take 1 tablespoon of coconut oil before bed to help soften bowel movements by the morning.

- Keep your feet up on a stool when sitting on the toilet. This helps keep your rectal area relaxed and makes for easier pushing.

- Drink water! Water not only keeps you hydrated but keeps you regular, as well.

- Keep up with your Kegels. Kegels help pump blood out of the engorged pelvic veins and help strengthen the muscles around the anus.

- Add an extra 10 milligrams of vitamin B_6, as well as a vitamin B complex, to your supplements. You can also take an extra 1,000 milligrams of vitamin C, which is vital for maintaining strength in the walls of blood vessels.

- Avoid long hours of sitting or standing. Moving around keeps blood circulating throughout your system and keeps your blood vessels from swelling.

- Apply ice packs or crushed ice to your perineal area. You can also alternate using ice with warm compresses.

- Take one to six sociable garlic pearls a day. Sociable garlic doesn't affect your breath but gives you all the benefits of garlic.

- Insert a peeled clove of garlic into your rectum at night. Garlic can decrease itching and inflammation related to hemorrhoids.

- Apply live yogurt to the area. The bacteria from live yogurt help fight infection, and regular application of yogurt offers pain relief and reduces itching. Since yogurt is kept in the fridge, it also has a cooling effect on hemorrhoids. Aloe vera works similarly. You can buy aloe vera gel or keep an aloe plant in your home. Break off part of a leaf and squeeze out the gel.

- Soak four figs in hot water overnight and eat them in the morning. Figs are a natural laxative and can help prevent constipation. Continue this for 3 to 4 weeks.

- Chamomile and nettle leaf both keep inflammation down. You can drink them both in tea form.

- Apply comfrey root ointment to the hemorrhoids. Comfrey contains high levels of allantoin, which helps to speed up the natural replacement of healthy body cells. Comfrey is also a natural anti-inflammatory.

- Apply baking soda to hemorrhoids to reduce itching. You can apply baking soda wet or dry, as well as take a warm bath with baking soda sprinkled in the water.

- Blend two raw potatoes into liquid form and spread the mixture into a gauze bandage. Fold the bandage in half and apply to hemorrhoids for 5 to 10 minutes. The potato will work as an astringent and will soothe pain.

- Acupuncture can also help with hemorrhoids. Acupuncturists will use acupuncture points far from the anus (such as the top of the head or the calves) to draw energy away from the anus and stimulate circulation to the affected area.

YOGA FOR HEMORRHOIDS

These poses help take the pressure off, relax the body, and aid in circulation.

SUPPORTED FISH POSE

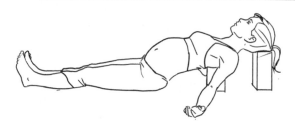

Lie flat on your back and place a medium block along your bra strap (between your shoulder blades), lifting your heart toward the sky. Extend your legs straight out in front of you and relax your feet. Place a high block under your head. Your arms should fall out at your sides with palms facing up, allowing your shoulders to drop open. Hold the pose for 1 minute.

CHILD'S POSE WITH BOLSTER

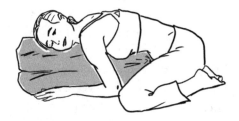

Get on the floor in a kneeling position, on all fours. Bring your big toes together but keep your knees far enough apart to make room for your belly. Place a bolster and/or folded blankets in between your thighs. Exhale and bring your body forward, lying over the padding. Make sure your entire trunk—from belly to head—is supported by the bolster or blankets. You can also put a folded blanket between your butt and heels for added support. Relax and hold the pose for 3 to 5 minutes.

FINDING BALANCE

"Change is the only constant."

—Heraclitus

The only thing that's certain in life is change. Yet oftentimes we cling in fear so tightly to our comfort zone and what we have outgrown that we have a hard time letting go and rolling with change. Every time we birth something new and reach a new level in life, there is always some type of death or a letting go that happens. This is a law of the universe.

I don't know about you, but I find that when I finally get into a groove and find balance—*boom!*—my life takes a turn and things start to shift. Change is inevitable. Personally, I have no intention of staying stuck or not growing in my life. Instead of clinging to the old, I ride the waves and go where the current of life is pulling me. I believe when you stop, look, and listen, you can see the signs that point you in the direction you're supposed to be going.

With this birth, and your new motherhood, will come a new way of looking, being, and feeling about life. So many things that mattered before won't matter as much anymore, and things you never gave two thoughts to might just become a major focus in your life. Change also comes with a restructuring of the way we manage our time and energy and find balance. As your life changes, you'll constantly have to readjust your energy—and time—to not only support your needs, but the needs of others, as well.

When you can truly live this concept, I promise it will save you *a lot* of anxiety down the road. Parenting is a great example— your baby is going to grow and evolve so fast. Just when you think you've mastered one stage of babyhood and what your child needs, he's on to a new phase. You must adapt and be flexible in order to roll with the changes.

Letting go of control and learning to ride the waves of life, the twists and turns, the highs and lows—without attachment— that's where you'll find peace. A great thing to remember is that life is always changing, and nothing ever stays the same. If things are hard or challenging, I always remind myself this is just how they are *right now*. It diffuses the energy and allows me to not be overly attached to my feelings or have my life remain stuck in a certain way.

There is a natural ebb and flow in life. I think about this often in labor as I help women ride the waves of their contractions. There is always a beginning and end, a high point and a low point. Life can become stressful when we don't go where its natural current is pulling us. When we fight against the natural flow, it's like swimming upstream in a roaring river, which will leave us totally depleted and exhausted. When you can surrender completely to the process or journey and become one with the waves, you will get there faster and easier than when you resist.

FINDING BALANCE CIRCLE

This is an exercise I do when change takes place in my life. I also like trying this with my clients, especially new moms. It's not difficult, but it will open your eyes to how your life is structured at the moment and hopefully give you some clarity about where you are now and where you may want to go.

1. Draw a big circle on a piece of paper.

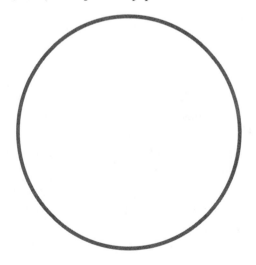

2. Pretend you're slicing a pie. Slice out of the circle the amount of time and energy you spend on:

- Your job/career
- Your relationship
- Your family
- Fun/social activities/ friends/recreation
- Health/self-care
- Financial matters
- Alone time or downtime/ relaxation

3. Take a look at your sliced circle/pie. Notice what's out of balance, what you need more of, or what slices are exactly the right size. Next, grab your calendar or computer and start listing or scheduling what you need to do to have more balance in your life. This will change weekly or monthly, as some days and times might be busier than others. Like I said before, the ebb and flow of life are constant. During both your calm and busy times, keeping things in balance will allow for a more peaceful ride.

"PLUCKING OUT THE WEEDS" MEDITATION

"Energy is contagious, positive and negative alike. I will forever be mindful of what and who I am allowing into my space."

—Alex Elle

I love doing this meditation with my clients at this point in their pregnancies. Just like you need to keep your calendar in balance and make space for what's important in your life, you need to take stock of habits, people, and activities that are *not* impacting your life in a positive way.

Get in a comfortable position and close your eyes. Begin to go within by taking four slow breaths in and four slow breaths out. If your mind starts to drift, bring it back to your breath. Scan your body and notice where you are tight. Send the breath into this area and exhale it out, allowing the breath to massage away the tension.

When you're feeling grounded and more relaxed, start to scan your life as if you're watching a movie. See yourself standing in the middle of your life, and begin to notice who and what is all around you.

- Do you feel happy and content with the people and things you surround yourself with?

- Do these things and people you spend time with feed you or deplete you?

- Are any toxic behaviors, patterns, habits, or thoughts holding you back from being the best version of yourself?

- Take a look at your home—all of the rooms, closets, and spaces. Is there clutter and stuff just lying around, taking up space?

Notice what comes up for you. Now, just like a gardener pulls weeds out of a garden, begin to pluck out of your life what needs to go, what's holding you back or wasting space in your life. You can also imagine a big vacuum sucking out anything that no longer serves you or isn't healthy for you anymore.

Now, feel yourself in the new space you've made. Do you feel lighter and have more breathing room? You might want to meditate on and feel the space. Notice if anything intuitively pops in. Start to think about what you want to fill this new-found space with.

- What kind of people do you want to play with?

- How do you want to start showing up for yourself and others?

- Where and with whom do you want to spend your time and energy?

- How does your home look and feel without all the clutter taking up space?

Imagine all the beautiful new parts of your life sprouting up from the ground all around you.

*"Let us reflect on what is truly of value in life,
what gives meaning to our lives, and set our
priorities on the basis of that."*

—the 14th Dalai Lama

Lactation Nutrition

This superquick, highly nutritious oatmeal recipe is a huge favorite with my clients. It makes for a power-packed breakfast that gives you tons of energy, helps increase your breast milk production, and calms your nerves as well as boosts your mood.

1 package organic quick oats

Vanilla almond milk (equal to amount of water on package directions)

½ banana, sliced

1 handful of raisins

⅓ cup sliced almonds

1 tablespoon honey

Pinch of Himalayan sea salt

Cook the desired serving size of oats according to the directions on the package. But instead of water, substitute vanilla almond milk. After the oats are cooked, lower the heat to a simmer and add the banana, raisins, almonds, honey, and salt. Add more almond milk during cooking if the oatmeal is too thick.

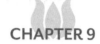

CHAPTER 9

Month Nine

LIVING IN JOY

"Appreciation is a doorway into your heart, it opens your heart and allows you to experience more love in your life."

—**Sanaya Roman**

When you look back on your childhood, what are some of your fondest memories? Maybe they are of great times with your friends at school, adventures with siblings, or valuable time spent with grandparents. For many of us, some of the best memories from childhood are of times when our parents were happy and engaged with us.

Now it's your turn to be the parent! How do you envision spending time with your baby? Do you see long afternoons at the playground, time together at a park, quiet time reading or playing games before bed? Raising a child will be one of the most joyful, rewarding, fulfilling, and challenging things you'll ever experience.

This chapter focuses on living in joy and finding gratitude and acceptance that you can carry throughout your life.

In a few short weeks, you'll finally meet your baby. This is such an exciting part of pregnancy. However, it's also a time when you might start feeling a bit more physically uncomfortable. Your back and hips might ache. Or your feet might swell. Or you might not be sleeping well. These inconveniences and discomforts might be starting to wear on you. I always tell my clients, "When you finally see this baby of yours, you won't remember any of this!" And all the sleepless nights of nonstop peeing and tossing and turning are actually preparing you for life with a newborn.

"Worry is a misuse of your imagination."
—Unknown

Coming toward the end of your pregnancy can also bring up a lot of fears. Around now, this whole "I'm having a baby" thing is definitely more of a reality, and that can cause some unexpected anxiety. When I prep my clients for birth, one of the sessions we do right before birth works through fears they might have about labor, birth, or being a mother. During labor, things can sometimes unexpectedly stall or even stop. I always have my clients change position regularly (by walking, kneeling, sitting on a birth ball, rocking on all fours, and so on)—anything that allows gravity to help the baby corkscrew down into the pelvis. If labor stalls and my clients need a rest, I use this time to give them a break. Otherwise, the first thing I would change is the position they are in. If that doesn't get it going again, I'll ask them if they are feeling okay, fearful, or worried about anything. Getting my clients to talk about whatever is worrying them allows that emotion to be released and usually gets things moving again.

I once worked with a woman who was very religious. Part of her religion was the belief that you don't buy anything for the baby or get the nursery ready until after the baby is born. It's a superstition that nothing should be done to acknowledge a baby is coming until it's out of the womb, just in case something happens. This woman's labor was going great—until, all of a sudden, it completely stalled. I tried massage, relaxation breathing, and visualizations and put her in different positions. Still, nothing was happening. I then asked her if she was worried about anything.

My client looked blankly at me—and then burst into tears! She explained that she felt completely unprepared for the arrival of her baby. Her house wasn't in order for a newborn and she didn't have anything she felt she needed for the baby. I assured her that right after birth, all the baby needs is her. I then asked what she needed right away. I wrote everything she told me in an e-mail and promised her that as soon as the baby was born I would send the e-mail out, asking friends and family to pick up what she needed. This shifted everything. My client relaxed, was able to let go, and her labor started again. A few hours later, she birthed a healthy baby.

It's difficult to feel safe about the unknown. If you're a first-time mother, thinking about giving birth and motherhood can be scary, as is anything you haven't done before. Even if this isn't your first baby, the thought of labor and delivery, and starting life with another baby, can bring on anxiety.

"In addition to showing gratitude to others, place emphasis on showing gratitude to yourself."
—Doreen Virtue

When I start working with a mom-to-be, I ask her to write out a list of anything about birth or parenthood she may be worried, scared, nervous, or anxious about. I have dads and partners do this, too! I take this information and build my birth plan around what I can do to make them feel safe in labor. (We'll discuss birth plans in the next chapter.) Everyone has different fears—no two women are alike, and no two birth experiences are the same.

Here are some common anxieties you may relate to—and ways to relieve the stress they create.

Worrying about the due date. When I start working with someone, the first thing I do is have them let go of the attachment they have to their exact due date. Instead, I build a birth window for them. I've seen people go bananas if their babies don't come on their due dates. The current statistic is that only 4 percent of women actually deliver on their due date. New findings even say that due dates can vary by up to 5 weeks.

Take some of the pressure off yourself. Block out at least a week or even 10 days on each side of your estimated due date and trust that sometime in this birth window, your baby will be born. I live by this as well: When I'm on call for a birth, I start leaving my phone on 24/7 about 10 days before the due date and 10 days after the due date if the baby hasn't come yet. Here's another tip: Tack on an extra week or 10 days to the estimated due date your caregiver gives you and tell *that* date to all your friends and family. All the good-natured calls and texts to see if you're in labor yet can drive a mom-to-be crazy. Well-meaning friends and family are super excited for the arrival of your baby.

Not knowing when labor begins. At the end of pregnancy, you may wonder if every movement, ache, or pain means labor is starting. Some women experience very distinct signs of labor, while others do not. No one knows what causes labor to start or when it will begin, but several hormonal and physical changes may indicate the beginning of labor. These include:

- Water breaking
- A noticeable drop in your belly
- Passing of the mucus plug
- Consistent contractions
- Dilation of the cervix
- Soft stools

A good rule of thumb to measure labor is to use the 411 method: Contractions should be 4 minutes apart, lasting 1 minute, for at least 1 hour to consider yourself to be in active labor.

It can be very disappointing to get all excited that you are in labor only to find out it was false labor. Here's a trick to try: If your contractions are inconsistent or not progressing, try drinking two huge glasses of water, lying down on your side, and taking a catnap. If you're in true labor, your contractions won't stop, while in false labor, they will.

Not being able to handle the pain. Expressing fear about pain and discussing pain management are very important before you start labor. With my clients, I talk about and work with them on different pain management skills and exercises such as breathwork, meditation, movement, visualizations, and massage.

Pooping while pushing. I'm not going to lie—there's a major possibility that you're going to poop while pushing your baby out. Many times women don't even realize it's happening, and if it does, it's usually a very small amount. A doctor, midwife, or nurse will clean it up *very* quickly.

Having a Caesarean section. You may be having a planned C-section, or it may be unexpected. Either way, this is a very common worry. I advise my clients to read about how the procedure is performed and what risks and options they may have, as I believe staying well informed will make you less likely to panic over the unknown. You can also educate yourself on how to avoid having a C-section. This can include interviewing caregivers about when they would feel the need to perform a C-section, as well as their C-section percentage; finding a caregiver with a low C-section rate who is on the same page with you about your birth; and learning different birthing techniques for optimal fetal positioning, pain management techniques to help you along in labor, and options for a more natural childbirth. Make sure your caregiver is on your time and your baby's time, not her own time.

Having an episiotomy. An episiotomy is a surgical incision used to enlarge the vaginal opening to help deliver a baby. Again, I have my clients read about what it is and how it may affect them postbirth. I encourage them to perform perineal massage (see Chapter 8). Use a hot compress on the perineum or have a caregiver do perineal massage during the pushing phase. You can also breathe through contractions for a few breaths instead of pushing when your baby is crowning to allow the perineum to stretch on its own.

One of the best ways to avoid an episiotomy is to tell your caregiver that you don't want one and would like to avoid one if possible.

Not having the energy to last throughout labor. Labor is definitely a marathon, and it requires pacing, determination, and endurance. Labor can be a long process with ups and downs and different phases to experience. I encourage women to conserve their energy as much as possible, right from the beginning of labor. Depending on the time of day and a woman's energy level, labor can be started in different positions. If my client is tired, I recommend that she lie on her side with some pillows in between her legs to help open up the pelvis. If she has more energy, I have her walk around so gravity can help get the baby down. If I have someone on a birth ball, I might have her lean forward on some pillows and massage her back and head. I always make sure my clients rest and recharge in between contractions to help conserve their energy. Ask your partner, doula, or someone from your support team for a massage in between contractions. Also, always eat and drink throughout labor. Try to have a good meal before contractions really start and then a few bites here and there when you can. Women sometimes vomit during labor because of all the extra hormones in their bodies, so try to eat simple foods. Smoothies, yogurt, oatmeal, fruit, natural energy bars, and crackers are all great snacks (and won't be too disturbing if they come back up).

When you conserve your energy, you'll be better off in the long run. Trust in your natural instincts and the birth process, and that your body and baby know exactly what they're supposed to do.

Being around germs. Many women freak out about germs, especially right before and during the birth. If I know someone is nervous about germs, I go out of my way to make her feel safe. If she's having the baby in a hospital or birthing center, I have her bring slippers and her own clothes and bedding, if that makes her more comfortable. I make sure a bottle of hand sanitizer is ready when she needs it, and I check to make sure the bathroom is clean. As labor goes on, she'll usually forget about germs, but until that point it's important to feel safe enough to let go and allow labor to progress.

Having an uninvited family member come to the birth. As a doula, this is a question that comes up a lot when I prep a couple for the birth of a child. I always ask, "Do you really want so-and-so there?" It always amazes me how many people answer no and then say they feel guilty about their decision. I advocate acknowledging what truly feels right and then setting firm boundaries. Mixed messages can often result in an uncomfortable situation for everyone. I can't tell you how many mothers and mothers-in-law I've had to escort out of the delivery room.

The birth of your child may very well be one of the most important and exciting days of your life. Anyone that brings drama, causes stress, or is unsupportive, judgmental, or makes you uncomfortable should not be allowed in the delivery room. This is also not a time to mend a troubled relationship. Remember, it's your day— you have a right to have your birth experience be what you would like even if it might upset other people. Just remember, you can't please everyone all of the time. This is great practice for setting boundaries and saying no as a parent, too.

If you'd like to invite anyone to the birth, think about people you're close to who are nurturing, supportive, and loving and whom you trust to be a part of this experience. Speak with them

SURFACE SPRAY

This is a great homemade, naturally sourced spray for all surfaces. Mix it in a spray bottle, bring it to the hospital, and use it on the bed, chairs—anything you think needs to be refreshed. All three oils have antibiotic, antibacterial, antiviral, and antifungal properties.

- 1 cup water
- 20 drops lemon essential oil
- 20 drops eucalyptus oil
- 10 drops tea tree oil

before the birth about how they can best support you and what you might need from them. Both you and your partner need to be on the same page and support each other with this.

"Time is an illusion."

—Albert Einstein

YOUR CHANGING BODY

You are *so* close to meeting your baby. You may be experiencing insomnia and feeling more physically uncomfortable. This is also the time of much anticipation and impatience, a time of thinking about the person you've created and will finally get to hold in your arms. It is super easy to want this month to fly by, to meet your baby and begin the next phase of your life together. Take time to be joyful and find the gratitude in little things. The last 4 weeks of your pregnancy might be more physically challenging as your body is in constant motion to get ready for the main event.

Your breasts will first produce colostrum after you give birth, and you may even notice some colostrum now. Your milk is there and will be ready to flow a few days following birth. A hormone from your placenta, called prolactin, triggers milk production. When the placenta is delivered after the baby, prolactin will start the process of your milk "coming in," or "letting down."

Around the midpoint of pregnancy, your hands, feet, ankles, and even face may start to experience puffiness or swelling. This is called edema, and it's a very common part of pregnancy. What happens is that changes in blood chemistry cause fluid to shift into your tissues, and by the third trimester, the weight of your uterus puts so much pressure on your veins and the vena cava (the large vein on the right side of your body that carries blood from your legs and feet back up to your heart) that blood can pool, forcing fluid retention below the knees. Edema also comes with some discomfort, such as shoes or pants not fitting properly and a general swollen look that you're just not used to seeing.

Some ways to relieve the effects of edema include the following:

- Drink water! I can't stress enough how important it is to stay hydrated, especially to support your increased blood production and faster bloodflow.
- Prop up your feet when you can, to allow blood to flow away from your feet faster.
- Avoid crossing your ankles or feet when you sit. Crossing your legs inhibits bloodflow.
- Use cool compresses on your legs and ankles to get relief from swelling.
- Massage can work wonders on sore, swollen legs and feet.

By the end of this month, you'll probably feel some real relief from the baby pushing upward into your rib cage and lungs. During this month, your baby will "engage" or "drop" into your pelvis (2 to 3 weeks before delivery in first-time moms, closer to the due date in later pregnancies).

During the end of pregnancy, many of my clients complain of pelvic pain. This is one of the reasons why it's important to keep up with your Kegels throughout your pregnancy. My chiropractor, body mechanics genius Dennis Colonello, DC, PT, offered the following exercise to strengthen your pelvic floor: Stand with your feet facing forward a little wider than hip-distance apart. Imagine an earthquake that's splitting the earth in between your feet. Don't let your feet move apart! Instead, squeeze your butt and draw in your feet as if you're trying to drag the earth back together again. Hold that squeeze for 10 seconds, and release. Do this three times. This exercise will engage the pelvic floor and inner thighs.

YOUR GROWING BABY

During the ninth month, your baby can use his eyes to see clearly, use his ears to distinguish sounds, suck his thumb, and cover his face with his hands. He has put on fat and filled out, and his skin will be as smooth and soft as a newborn baby's. Every child is a different size at birth. At 40 weeks, most newborns weigh anywhere from 6 to 9 pounds and are 18 to 20 inches long. This is comparable to a small watermelon.

When the baby drops into your pelvis, its movement patterns will change yet again. You'll feel fewer kicks and more wiggles and turns. If your baby's head is engaged, every turn might feel like small, sharp twinges close to your cervix, a sign that he's getting ready to make his big debut. You still want to count movements, however, since it's important to feel something occurring at least every hour.

LABOR TAKES TIME

In the ninth month, labor is likely one of the biggest things on your mind. My clients always want to know how long labor will take, what the experience will be like, and when their baby will arrive. I know the end of pregnancy can be really uncomfortable. Of course, you can try to do things to help labor along, but just know and trust that your baby will come when your body and she are good and ready. There is a natural, divine timing to all things, and no one embodies this more than a newborn.

Remember: Labor takes time! This is especially true for first-time moms. The average labor for a first child is anywhere from 12 to 24 hours. Knowing that, it's important to pace yourself and manage your time and energy wisely. Remember my marathon analogy? You wouldn't run a marathon without practicing by running for months beforehand. You also wouldn't race without sleeping the night before and taking in food and water the day of the race. And you wouldn't use up all your energy at the start of the race, knowing you have a long way to run and that the last mile will require all your strength.

Take your time. Labor at home for as long as you can if you're planning on going to the hospital, and use your doula or partner to coach, support, and guide you so you can better ride the waves of each contraction. Try to rest as much as possible in between contractions. Stay hydrated and eat small meals and snacks (typically, hospitals restrict food during labor). Remember to breathe through any uncomfortable sensations. These are totally natural; it's just your body doing exactly what it's supposed to do.

Over the years, I've often found that women aren't allowed time to labor and give birth properly in conventional hospitals. It's different if you have a midwife or a home birth, but in hospitals I believe women need to be given more time. (Obviously, if there are any complications, it's a different story.) There is a natural, powerful force that we have as women that takes over in labor if you surrender and allow it in. It's this strength of the great mother who will do anything for her children. Remember, it isn't the caregiver's time to have a baby—it's yours! Don't let anyone rush the process, especially if you and your baby are holding steady and are doing great.

ATTITUDE AND GRATITUDE

"God gave you a gift of 86,400 seconds today. Have you used one to say thank you?"

—William Arthur Ward

One of the best ways to shift your energy from negative to positive is by bringing your attention to what you feel grateful for. You can't help but be in a good mood when you focus on what's

Fetuses move once a minute, on average, and their movements are remarkably similar to how newborns behave. They yawn, swallow, and make breathing motions. They suck their thumbs and play with their umbilical cords and other body parts. Near full term, fetuses even scrunch and stretch their mouths and noses into the same facial expressions that newborns make.

going right in your life instead of what's going wrong. People often tend to focus on what they *don't* have instead of on all their gifts. When your attention is on what's lacking, you will never feel fulfilled or satisfied. But when you begin to see all that you *do* have, your life becomes richer than you ever thought possible. Living in gratitude raises your vibration and brings more joy, and you begin to see abundance everywhere.

People with a strong sense of gratitude and appreciation don't necessarily have more than others; they simply see more beauty in their lives. Get your journal and write about everything that's bothering you. Let it rip for 2 minutes, and then stop. Without pausing to think, switch gears and write about everything that's going right in your life and what you're thankful for. Just as you switched gears in your writing here, you have the power to shift your attitude in a snap. You can shift your energy toward the positive any time you need to in your life.

If you ever feel as if something in your life isn't "enough," try practicing an attitude of thankfulness. You will start to realize how good your life really is. You can change your attitude from negative to positive just by living in gratitude. Just like we train our bodies in the gym, we can train our minds to go to the positive and find the gratitude in the moment. I once had a client who really didn't like being pregnant. I'm not going to lie—some women don't! She was uncomfortable, depressed, and aggravated. We did a session together one day that shifted everything for her. I told her that not everyone loves being pregnant and that's okay, but your baby feels this energy you emit. I then asked her if she was looking forward to being a mother and having this child. Her whole body softened and a smile formed on her mouth. She said she couldn't wait to love and hold this baby in her arms. I had her

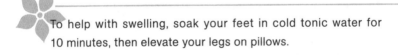

To help with swelling, soak your feet in cold tonic water for 10 minutes, then elevate your legs on pillows.

close her eyes and think about holding him in her arms and what her life with this child and her family would be like.

From this place, I had her breathe this feeling of joy and excitement into her heart, hold her belly, and say out loud how thankful she was to be a mother and that she couldn't wait to meet her baby. I also had her thank him for choosing her to be his mom and say how lucky she felt to get pregnant so easily and how strong and healthy she and her baby were. I had her do this daily, and it shifted the whole experience for her.

Love Soak Bath Meditation

Roses are the flowers of love, and rose oil calms and uplifts the spirit. Both grapefruit and geranium lift the spirit and act as antidepressants. Rose quartz is a stone of love and femininity. It brings love, peace, harmony, and joy. I hope you find this love bath and meditation calming, peaceful, and a special, quiet time between you and your baby-to-be.

2 rose quartz crystals

1 cup Dr. Bronner's Unscented Baby Mild Pure Castile Soap

20 drops rose oil

5 drops grapefruit oil

3 drops geranium oil

2 tablespoons dried crushed rose petals or a handful or two of fresh petals

Place the rose quartz crystals in the bathtub and draw a bath.

Mix the soap and rose, grapefruit, and geranium oils into the bath.

When the bath is full, throw in the flowers.

Get comfortable in the tub and use your left hand to place 1 rose quartz crystal on your heart and your right hand to place the other rose quartz crystal on your belly. Now, start the following meditation.

While sitting comfortably in the bath, imagine seeing yourself face-to-face with your baby. You can even imagine her in the bath with you. (Well, technically, she is.) Imagine placing your left hand on your heart and your right hand on hers. Take a deep breath into your heart and

(continued on page 223)

JOURNAL WORK:
PRACTICE LIVING IN GRATITUDE

*"If the only prayer you said was thank you,
that would be enough."*

—**Meister Eckhart**

We take for granted some of the most important things in our lives. It's when we feel gratitude for the simple things in life that we begin to see how lucky we really are. Whatever you acknowledge and appreciate will increase in your life. Starting today, let gratitude be your new attitude!

When you get a few moments, try one of these exercises.

- Look around your home. Silently acknowledge or write down five things about your home that you are thankful for.

- Look at your relationship. We're really good at telling the other person what he or she is doing wrong and don't spend enough time expressing what he or she is doing right. Quietly acknowledge or write down five things about your relationship with your partner or another loved one that you are grateful for. If you're single, list five positive things about being single.

- Think about your job. What are five things that you like about your career? If you aren't working right now, think about five things that you enjoy about not working.

- Consider your family. Write down or think about five things that you appreciate about your family.

- Every night before bed, silently acknowledge or write down five things you were grateful for that day. Also, tell your partner a few things you appreciate about him and/or something he did that day that you're thankful for.

Give thanks to yourself and acknowledge everything that makes you unique and special. Give thanks for your body and your health.

feel all the love and gratitude you have for this baby. Let that love beam out of your heart, through your hands, and into her heart. Now, begin to tell her how much you appreciate her and how having her in your life is a blessing, and why. Thank your baby for choosing you to be her mommy, and tell her how excited you are to meet her and raise her. Allow the love and gratitude to pour out of your heart, right into her heart, as well as the water that surrounds you.

When you're out of the tub, write out all of the love and gratitude that you felt in a letter to your baby. Think about your baby and how you can't wait to meet her, how grateful you are for her, and how much you appreciate her presence in your life. Finally, place this letter in an envelope somewhere safe where you'll remember where it is. Pick a future birthday or life event when you can gift her with this love letter.

You can also try doing this bath meditation with a focus on your partner (or anyone special in your life). Think about all the things you are grateful for, respect, and love about him. Think about how much you appreciate him and need him in your life. From this place of the heart, write a love letter to your partner and give it to him when it feels right to do so. He'll appreciate this more than you will ever know.

BODY AWARENESS BEFORE LABOR

Right now, as you're entering the final few weeks of your pregnancy, I'd really like you to become even more aware of your body—how it's feeling, how your baby is moving, any changes you may be experiencing. I prepare my clients for childbirth through yoga, breathwork, and visualization. I've walked you through all of these techniques throughout this book, so feel free to use them whenever you can. I believe that the more tuned-in and connected you are to your body and needs, the easier time you'll have navigating the waves of contractions during labor. If you resist or fight the sensation of discomfort, your body will tighten, contract, and hold on. In birth, resistance is counterintuitive to the process. Learning to surrender as you ride out the contractions will help your body let go, open up, and allow your baby to drop down.

Here are a few simple poses to help prepare your body and breathing for childbirth.

SIMPLE SEATED BREATHWORK

We've talked about this breathwork before, so you may be wondering why I'm having you do it again. In labor, when you breathe into your baby during a contraction, you're helping him by sending him extra oxygen and bloodflow. As you relax on the exhalation, your body is able to open up more and your baby can corkscrew his way down to the birth canal. During a client's labor, I'll also place my hand on her belly during a contraction and say, "Breathe into my hand and, as you exhale, let everything relax." By softening your body, you're helping your baby so much! He'll be able to more easily drop down and make his way out and into your arms.

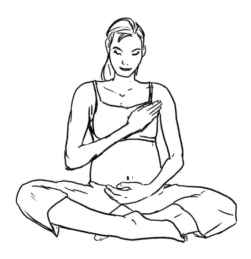

Sit in a cross-legged position and place your right hand on your heart and your left hand on your belly. (Intuitively find your baby with your left hand.) Through your nose, slowly breathe in four deep breaths, directing them right into your heart. Send that breath down to your baby. Exhale slowly through your mouth as your shoulders, jaw, belly, and whole body relax. Do this a few times. Next, inhale through your nose the word "Let" and exhale through your mouth "go," softening and relaxing everything on the exhale. Next breathe in the word "I" and exhale the word "surrender." Lastly, breathe in "Body" and then exhale "relaxes."

WAG THE TAIL

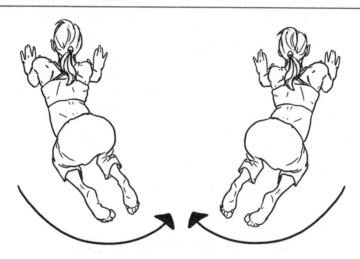

Get on all fours, with your hands flat on the floor under your shoulders and your knees on the floor, hip-distance apart. Begin to slowly rock your hips from side to side like you're rocking your baby in a cradle. Breathe in through your nose and into your baby and exhale through your mouth, again letting your belly drop and relax. I usually place my hand under my client's belly here and have her breathe into my hand again. As she exhales, I say, "Let your belly go as your baby drops into my hand." This pose is great to relax your belly. As women, we constantly grip our bellies when we're stressed or nervous, but you don't want to do this during labor. This pose helps relax the area and, again, will help you in surrendering to (instead of fighting) the contraction.

Later on in pregnancy, hormones relax and soften the ligaments of the pelvic area. Your pelvis is not fused together and does open for the birth of your baby. Your baby's head is soft and moldable to fit in the birth canal.

The organization Spinning Babies helps women with fetal positioning through classes, videos, and online tutorials (with help from a midwife or caregiver). One way it suggests moms-to-be may have success turning a breech baby (a baby not in a head-down position) is in a swimming pool. The method involves doing handstands in water that comes up to the tops of the thighs. The theory is that by going upside-down and doing an inversion, the extra buoyancy of the baby in water helps bring her away from the pelvis, allowing her to reposition herself. For more information about turning breech babies, I highly recommend the Spinning Babies Web site (www.spinningbabies.com).

GET YOUR LABOR GOING!

"There is a secret in our culture, and it's not that birth is painful. It's that women are strong."

—Laura Stavoe Harm

You can help get your labor moving along by stimulating the energy of the 2nd chakra (reproductive area). Activities that help release oxytocin, the hormone released both in labor and in love, help get things moving. Here's my short list of ways to prep your body and jump-start your labor. I usually have my clients do the following a month before their estimated due date.

- Have sex, sex, and even more sex! Having orgasms helps relax you and releases oxytocin.

- Keep doing your squats! The movement can strengthen your pelvic floor and help bring baby's head down, which puts pressure on the cervix and helps with dilation.

- Try nipple stimulation, either by hand or with a breast pump. This encourages your body to start contractions by simulating a nursing baby, which also releases oxytocin.

- Try walking, walking, more walking, even marching and dancing. Gravity and movement can stimulate your cervix and trigger oxytocin release.

- With your legs straddling a birth ball, bounce hard up and down.

- Eat spicy food. Spices stimulate your stomach, which in turn can stimulate your uterus, triggering labor.

- Eat pineapple and figs. These fruits contain the enzyme bromelain, which is thought to help soften your cervix and bring on labor. You can also take bromelain capsules.

- Burn clary sage oil in an aromatherapy diffuser, or place 40 drops in a bath and soak for 20 minutes, or rub a few drops on your belly. The clary sage causes uterine contractions, which can help bring on labor.

- Get acupuncture on labor-inducing pressure points.

- Deeply massage the backs of your heels. This is one pressure point on your foot that can stimulate labor.

- Drink a few cups of raspberry leaf tea daily to strengthen and tone your uterus.

- Take primrose oil either orally or vaginally to help soften your cervix.

If all else fails, keep meditating and breathing using the "Let go" techniques I've taught you throughout the book. Surrender to the process, trusting that your baby will come when it's good and ready. Enjoy your free and alone time and rest while you can because right around the corner you are going to be *very* busy taking care of your new baby.

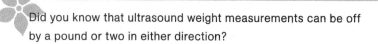

Did you know that ultrasound weight measurements can be off by a pound or two in either direction?

WHAT'S IN YOUR HOSPITAL BAG?

If you're planning to give birth at a hospital or birthing center, prepare early and have your hospital bag packed in advance just in case you go into labor earlier than expected. Have the bag by your front door or garage, so you can grab it and go when it's time! Here's what you should pack.

For the Hospital or Birthing Center

- **Birth plan.** (See Chapter 10.) Make a few copies—one for you, one for your caregiver, and one for the hospital or birthing center.

- **Essential documents.** Insurance card, hospital forms, list of people to contact when the baby is born, and, if you're planning on banking cord blood, the cord blood kit and papers.

- **Birth ball.** Sitting upright on a birth ball allows your baby's head to push on your cervix, which helps you dilate. You can sit on it, bounce, rock from side to side, do hip circles, make figure eights, squat against it, and lean against the wall on it.

- **Eyeglasses.** You may not want to deal with contact lenses while in labor, so wear your glasses to the hospital or have them ready.

- **Relaxation items.** Earplugs, sleep mask, white noise machine, calming or meaningful music, flameless candles, aromatherapy oils and electric diffuser. These all help you relax.

- **Arnica tablets.** Take one tube of arnica tablets every 4 hours during birth and after to speed up healing.

Only 1 in 10 women's water breaks before labor begins. Most women's water breaks just before the second stage of labor (the pushing stage), when they are nearly fully dilated.

- **Colace.** This is a stool softener to help prevent constipation after giving birth.

- **Inspirational objects.** Crystals, photos of loved ones or gurus, affirmations.

- **Massage cream.** So your partner can massage you during labor.

- **Nightgown and/or bathrobe.** The hospital has gowns for laboring women, but you are allowed to wear your own. Bring something loose, breathable, and short-sleeved (so the nurse can take your blood pressure). Make sure it's something you won't feel bad about throwing away afterward.

- **Slippers or flip-flops.** You can wear socks but, if you're planning on walking around during labor, slippers or flip-flops provide better support. These will also be helpful during your stay at the hospital after birth.

- **Whatever will help comfort you.** Bring what you need to keep you comfortable! This includes your own pillow, cozy blanket, music, photos of loved ones or a place that centers you, or anything else you find reassuring and calming.

For Your Partner/Labor Coach

- **Electronic devices.** Make sure the camera, video camera, phone, iPad, iPod, speakers, computer, and so on are fully charged; and don't forget to pack your chargers.

- **Toiletries.** Your partner should be prepared for an overnight stay as well, so have him or her bring a toothbrush and toothpaste, comb or brush, deodorant, hair products, etc.

- **Change of clothes.** Have your partner pack a change of clothes so he or she can feel fresh. Make sure he or she brings something to keep warm, as hospitals tend to be chilly.

- **Money.** For hospit al parking, vending machines, or other food from the hospital.

HOME BIRTH PACKING LIST

If you are preparing for a home birth, your midwife may have you purchase a birth kit either through her or online. The midwife may provide a birthing pool, but if she doesn't, you can use your bathtub, buy an inflatable kiddie pool, or order a birthing pool online at yourwaterbirth.com.

The midwife may also bring a birthing stool. I always suggest getting a birth ball, which you can use while you are in labor.

The following items are other birthing supplies you will need:

Large stack of clean washcloths and towels

Waterproof mattress cover

Plastic tarp to go under the pool

Plastic sheets to protect the floor and furniture

Clean sheets for the bed (old ones or a set that you don't mind getting stained)

Large bowl or container for the placenta

Box of large, heavy-duty trash bags

Hose that is long enough to fill up the tub

Receiving blankets for the baby

Heating pad, hot water bottle, or rice pack that you can heat

Ice pack

Bucket or pot in case you need to vomit

Massage cream and or oil

After You Deliver

- **Another nightgown** or other pajamas.
- **Contact list.** For your big e-mail announcement, text, or phone calls!

You will already be in the comfort of your own home, but you may want to make it even more comfortable and create a peaceful vibe by adding the following:

Candles

Aromatherapy

Music

Also, stock up on easy-to-digest snacks and drinks, including:

Yogurt

Oatmeal bars

Fruit

Applesauce

Smoothies

Natural peanut butter and jelly sandwiches

Water

Coconut water

Lori B's Fabulously Yummy LaborAde (see pages 235–236)

Ice chips (Laboring women tend to run hot, so you can use the ice in drinks or to suck on. It also feels good to place the ice on the back of the neck or forehead.)

🖎 **Toiletries.** Toothbrush and toothpaste, deodorant, hairbrush, shampoo, soap, moisturizer, any personal items you use from home.

🖎 **Nursing bras, breast pads, and nipple cream.**

🖎 **Maternity underwear.** Hospitals provide mesh underwear, but you'll probably be more comfortable in your own underwear. The hospital will provide sanitary pads because you'll still bleed after delivery. Make sure you have a supply of heavy-duty pads waiting at home, too.

- **Journal.** You may not be ready to write down your entire birth story just yet, but it's helpful to have paper and pen handy for other notes or questions you may have. Write down the times your baby nurses or eats, thoughts and memories, and well-wishes from family and friends who visit.

- **Clean clothes to go home in.** Have a comfortable outfit for the ride home and those first moments back home with your baby.

For the Baby

- **Natural soap and lotion for bathing.** You'll get to choose whether to have your baby bathed or not after birth. If you want to, you can bring your own supplies and give them to the nurse.

- **A couple of changes of clothing.** Hospitals have plenty of blankets to wrap your baby in after birth, but you may want her to wear a simple newborn T-shirt as well. You may also want to bring a hat or socks for extra warmth. Many people also have a special "going home" outfit for when they leave the hospital.

- **Newborn-sized diapers.** The hospital will provide you with diapers while you're there, but it's always good to have extra on hand.

- **Infant car seat.** Babies aren't allowed to leave the hospital unless they're properly buckled into an infant car seat. Infant car seats can be tricky to set up and get the baby properly settled into without practice, so take some time and use a doll to learn how the seat works.

- **BPA-free pacifier,** if you choose to use one.

WHAT'S IN MY DOULA BAG?

Just like the hospital bag you're starting to pack, I also have what I call my doula "bag of tricks" I bring with me to every birth. Over the years I've gathered lots of helpful goodies to help with the birthing process. Every birth experience I've been part of has been different. I'm always learning what's helpful to women in labor, so I'm constantly adding new items to my repertoire. Of course, add any or all of them to your own bag.

- **Battery-operated, flameless candles.** Nothing creates a soothing atmosphere like candlelight, but you can't use an open flame in a hospital. These candles are a must to create a good, relaxing vibe.

- **Scent ball aromatherapy diffuser and essential oils.** As comfortable as a hospital will try to make you feel during labor and delivery, it's still a blah and stale environment. Adding some yummy-smelling oils will help shift the whole feeling in the room. I like to use oils of clary sage and lavender mixed together. As the birth progresses, I switch to a blend of ylang-ylang and sweet orange oils.

- **Spectrum organic unscented coconut oil.** I use this to massage my client's back, head, legs, and feet. I melt the oil and add a mix of eucalyptus, clary sage, and lavender oils. I also use another blend of lavender and sandalwood oils on the head to help relax and calm the mind.

- **Peppermint oil.** When my client starts to get tired, I dab a drop on each temple. It's an instant pick-me-up.

- **Earplugs.** Block out noise and, again, help clients achieve a deeper sleep.

- **Arnica 30x.** I feed it to my clients during labor and after to help with healing.

- **Ginger brew, ginger tea, or fresh ginger root.** Helps to ease nausea.

- **Nux vomica.** Homeopathic remedy to help with nausea.

- **Red raspberry leaf tea.** Helps tone and strengthen the uterus and helps with pain.

- **Chamomile tea.** To help the mom (and others!) relax.

- **Honey.** For the tea and also for an energy boost.

- **Lollipops.** For a little extra energy and to help with dry mouth.

- **Ice bag.** For my clients' foreheads, to help cool them off.

- **Superfood bars, almonds, dried fruit, coconut water.** To munch on and drink.

- **Rescue Remedy.** This is a Bach Flower remedy that helps ease the nerves and calm you down. Believe it or not, I bring it for my pregnant clients but end up giving it to other people in the room, instead. I also have in my bag, just in case, Bach Flower remedies of olive (helps restore energy when you are physically and mentally exhausted), cherry plum (helps you act rationally and think clearly when you fear losing control), and white chestnut (encourages a peaceful and calm mind when worries come into your head).

- **The powdered drink Natural Calm.** I've mentioned this calcium-magnesium drink a few times in the book. It helps relax the body and mind. I bring this with me to make drinks for the birthing mama and anyone else in the room who may be feeling worried or stressed (partner, friends, parents, and in-laws). Remember: The calmer everyone in the room is, the calmer the laboring mother will be.

- **Sleep mask.** A sleep mask helps darken the room to promote sleep.

- **Hairbrush.** Sometimes, epidurals cause itchiness. I use this to gently scratch my client's skin, and it works wonders.

- **Lip balm.** Keeps lips from getting dry.

- **Mints.** Freshen breath and help with dry mouth or nausea.

- **Rosewater face mist.** Misting water is soothing, refreshing, and a nice pick-me-up.

- **Paper or battery-operated fan.** Labor can make women hot.
- **Stress ball.** For my clients to squeeze during contractions.
- **Heating pad.** For back pain.
- **Fully loaded iPad or iPod and speakers,** with soothing relaxation music and sounds. I love kundalini chanting, ocean sounds, Reiki music, or spa music.

Start taking or inserting evening primrose oil during your last month of pregnancy. This oil contains prostaglandins, known to thin out the cervix so it can dilate easier and thus possibly encourage labor to start sooner. Start at Week 37: Either swallow one capsule a day or poke a hole in the capsule and insert it vaginally, placing it right up by the cervix. Each week, increase the amount: Week 38, take or place two capsules; Week 39, do three. By Week 40, you should be up to four capsules per day.

Lori B's Fabulously Yummy LaborAde

I usually make this for all my clients the minute I show up for their birth. I have them drink it throughout the whole birth process and afterward.

1 red raspberry leaf tea bag. Red raspberry leaf tea strengthens and tones the uterus. It also helps with bleeding during delivery and aids in production of breast milk.

1 nettle leaf tea bag. Nettle leaf tea is a natural muscle relaxer and is high in vitamin K to prevent hemorrhaging during delivery.

1 chamomile leaf tea bag. Chamomile tea relaxes the nerves, soothes labor pains and cramping, helps relieve nausea, and helps wounds heal faster.

1 teaspoon Natural Calm drink with added calcium (raspberry-lemon or orange flavor). This drink helps promote relaxation and soothes aching muscles.

Small pinch of Himalayan sea salt. Himalayan sea salt regulates fluid levels, restores electrolyte balance, and actually increases hydration.

It also prevents muscle cramping, lowers blood pressure, improves circulation, and improves mental clarity and mood.

Honey to taste. Honey provides energy from natural sugars.

Boil a pot of water. When it's boiling, take the pot off the stove. Add the raspberry leaf tea bag, nettle leaf tea bag, and chamomile leaf tea bag. Steep for about 7 minutes, then add the Natural Calm, sea salt, and honey. Drink hot or cold throughout labor.

FOODS FOR THE FUTURE

There's so much to think about in order to prepare your home, your family, and yourself for the arrival of your little one. Another important element of preparation happens in your kitchen—it's helpful to stock up on healthy foods and easy-to-make meals for you, your partner, and anyone else who may be there with you.

During this month, think about prepping food that can be frozen and then easily reheated. This can be anything from casseroles to soup to individually wrapped chicken breasts or hamburgers. You and your partner are going to be totally focused on the new baby, so it's great to have ready-to-go meals that are cost-effective and efficient, You can also start a file of menus from healthy restaurants in your area for takeout or delivery.

My mom makes this amazing lasagna that I share with all of my clients. It's hearty, healthy, and freezes perfectly. It makes enough to feed a group of people or provide a couple of meals for you and your partner. Pair it with a big green salad and enjoy.

My Mama's Lasagna

1 box (10 ounces) brown rice lasagna noodles

3 tablespoons olive oil, divided

1 clove garlic, diced

½ pound organic ground turkey

Salt, pepper, and garlic powder to taste

1 package (8 ounces) frozen organic spinach, thawed

1 package (8 ounces) sliced mushrooms

1 container (8 ounces) organic ricotta cheese

1 jar (24 ounces) organic marinara sauce

Grated Parmesan cheese to taste

A handful or two shredded organic mozzarella cheese

In a large pot, cook the noodles according to package directions, adding 1 tablespoon of the olive oil to prevent sticking. Meanwhile, preheat the oven to 375°F.

In a medium saucepan, cook the garlic in 1 tablespoon of the olive oil for 3 minutes, stirring frequently. Add the ground turkey and cook, stirring frequently, until no longer pink. Add the salt, pepper, and garlic powder, spinach, and mushrooms. Cook, stirring frequently, for 5 minutes.

In a medium bowl, combine the ricotta cheese with the ground turkey, spinach, and mushroom mixture. Mix well.

Coat the bottom of a 13" x 9" baking pan with the remaining 1 tablespoon of olive oil. Add a layer of marinara sauce, a layer of cooked noodles, and a layer of the ricotta mixture. Sprinkle Parmesan cheese on top. Top with a layer of mozzarella cheese. Repeat the layers of sauce, noodles, ricotta mixture, Parmesan, and mozzarella cheese until you run out of noodles and filling. Top everything with more sauce, then sprinkle mozzarella and Parmesan cheese on top.

Cover the pan with aluminum foil and bake for 35 minutes. Take the foil off and bake for another 10 minutes.

This also tastes great as a vegetarian version, so feel free to leave out the turkey and substitute different veggies.

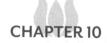

CHAPTER 10

LABOR, BIRTH, AND BEYOND

GO WITH THE FLOW

"The moment a child is born, the mother is also born. She never existed before. The woman existed, but the mother, never. A mother is something absolutely new."

—Unknown

This chapter tackles what many women think about for the entire pregnancy: preparing for the grand finale, the labor and birth, and getting to meet your baby! There are many options for how and where to birth your baby. Choosing the way you give birth is an individual and personal decision. This chapter will help you find the birth that's right for you. By creating a birth plan, you're laying out how you would like your baby's birth to be handled. Birth plans are also a great tool to educate you about all of your options and choices. If you don't state your needs, and you're planning on birthing in a hospital, the hospital staff will just follow protocol.

I encourage my clients to learn about all the different birth options throughout labor and afterward, such as getting an epidural versus having an unmedicated birth, having a home birth or a hospital birth, and so on. It's important to know your options—that you have choices and a *voice* about the way you want both you and your child treated and how you would like your birth to be handled.

A person who wants to run a marathon wouldn't just wake up one day and go run 26.2 miles—she would train for the big day. Well, birth is like that, too. Every meditation and journaling activity in this book helps prepare you for one of the most memorable days you'll ever have in your life—the day you get to birth and meet your child and yourself as a mother! The themes I gave you each month have given you tools to better navigate being a leader and parent for your child.

There are many different ways to birth a child. In order to plan for a labor and birth that you're comfortable with, you

STAY OUT OF THE FEAR ZONE

I once saw this quote: "Keep your negative birth stories to yourself: Both my baby and I are listening." As I explained in Chapter 9, fear shuts down your body and can stall labor. You'll undoubtedly hear birth stories of all kinds while you're pregnant. People love to share their experiences—the good, the bad, and the ugly. People will project the way they delivered their baby and think it should be the same for you. Let them know, politely, that you're focusing on the positive and not interested in the fear zone. Ask for their support and trust as you make your own decisions.

have to be honest with yourself. Just because your best friend had a totally natural, easy labor and delivery doesn't mean you'll have the same experience; conversely, just because a friend had a difficult or challenging birth doesn't mean the same thing will happen to you. Every woman is different, and in labor that means that women will have different pain thresholds, strengths and weaknesses, intentions and wills. It's awesome to be inspired by others, but labor and delivery are not a competitive sport!

TRUST THE PROCESS

"I am learning to trust the journey even when I do not understand it."

—-Mila Bron

You have a lot of choices to make about your labor and delivery. You may think you have all of the whos, whats, wheres, whens, and hows perfectly figured out. However, the birth journey is something you can't predict. Each and every birth unfolds in its own unique way.

Preparing for labor isn't just about planning details such as where you'll deliver and who will be with you. It's also about trusting yourself and the process of birth; having a plan and a good support team; and preparing to work toward your goal while allowing some flexibility in the process. Focus on yourself and do the best you can. In the end, I believe children come into this world how and when they are supposed to. Trust the process and the pace of your unique labor in order to stay healthy, calm, and centered.

Sometimes it helps to remind my clients that there *is* an end— labor is just the final part to get through. Before you know it, you'll get to meet your baby and hold him in your arms. Practice feeling gratitude for your strength and bask in this miracle of what your body is doing in making, housing, and birthing a baby.

WORK THE WABI-SABI

Wabi-sabi is a Japanese worldview that accepts imperfection as natural and beautiful and embraces finding this beauty in the imperfections all around you. Wabi-sabi asks you to look at the "imperfections" of things, such as their asymmetry, simplicity, or roughness, and to find the beauty in their imperfections. In life, perfection is an unattainable bar that you will never reach. Constantly striving for it will make you suffer.

Once, while hiking, my mom and I had a conversation about her pregnancy with me and my birth—they weren't exactly what one might call perfect. But in the end, that experience led me to my work as a pregnancy coach and doula. Those experiences were stepping-stones that established me and my path in the world today.

Sometimes, even if things don't seem perfect, when you look closer, there are moments of greatness within. That's finding the wabi-sabi in everything, finding perfection in the imperfection.

I have never seen or worked with the same two pregnant women, births, babies, or families. Everyone is unique. It makes me crazy when others project their ways onto another or put her down because she's doing something differently than they did. These people are not you, nor will they ever be. We all have our own unique strengths and weaknesses that make us the perfect parent, partner, or friend. The more you know who you are and accept it, the easier it will be to appreciate others' individuality and, ultimately, the better able you will be to accept your children for who they are as well.

CREATING YOUR BIRTH PLAN

I personally like to refer to creating a birth "intention" instead of a "plan" since, to me, a plan is set in stone with little wiggle room to change things without stress. Birth is karmic—you can have all the plans in the world, but sometimes things don't go the way you intended them to. By practicing nonattachment and trusting the process, you'll have more flexibility if you get pulled in a different

JOURNAL WORK: FINDING PERFECTION IN IMPERFECTION

Try this simple exercise:

- First, make a list of all the qualities that you like about yourself: your strengths, talents, anything that makes you unique and special.

- Now, make a list of the aspects of yourself that you don't feel are your best qualities.

Can you make any connections between the two lists? Or see how they balance each other out to make up your complete self? Good always comes with bad, light with darkness. Good and bad are part of the natural balance of the universe, as well as our selves. You may find these parts of yourself that you don't like in your children someday. When you can better accept them in yourself, you'll be better able to accept them in your children if they happen to possess the same energy. I myself know a certain sadness in life; it isn't something I like about myself or am proud of. By knowing this sadness is part of me and accepting it, I am more empathetic if a certain sadness comes up with someone around me. My sadness makes me more vulnerable, compassionate, and real. So what I find imperfect about myself really is perfect, especially in my line of work!

This month, think about the areas in your life or aspects of yourself that you don't feel are perfect. See if you can find the perfection (the beauty) in the imperfection. Start noticing the wabi-sabi all around you! A good example of wabi-sabi is found in the cracks, crevices, and textures that make aged wood interesting. Or look in an older woman's face and find the beauty in her wrinkles and laugh lines.

Also notice: What or whom are you competing with? What is this image of perfection you are trying to live up to? Is this image even realistic for you? Did someone project it onto you? If so, whose ideals are these? Are these people really like who you truly are? There is no one right way to do anything, but there is a right and perfect way for you, your children, and your family.

direction. This is a great metaphor for life in general and will help you with your parenting skills down the road as well! There will be times where life throws you a curveball. If you're overly focused on or attached to one rigid plan, you might miss the natural flow or the pull of the current guiding you along. When you try to control a situation, you hold on and become rigid, which tightens and hardens your body and energy—something you definitely don't want during labor.

Create your intention well ahead of time (use the guide on page 282) and know your options. State your needs, prepare for them, do the work, and then do your best to let go. Practice going with the flow and think about how you'll allow your birth to

JOURNAL WORK: GETTING YOUR FEARS OUT

"Believe you can and you're halfway there."
—Unknown

Fear is a big part of why many women cannot let go and relax during birth. Let's get all your fears out now before that process even begins! Grab a piece of paper (or a stack) and write out all your fears and worries about birth or being a mother or parent. Let it rip! Get it all out of your head and onto paper. Then look at this list and expand on it by writing out things you can do either now or during your birth to make yourself feel safe.

Now write about your ideal birth, almost like you are writing out a fairy tale. Write about what your perfect birth feels like. Who is there with you, what are their roles, and what are they doing to support you? What's the energy of the room like? How do you want to feel—calm and in the know? Then plan on playing soft music and bringing flameless candles or a plug-in aromatherapy diffuser and filling the air with some calming lavender oil. Or, if you're hoping the mood is light and fun, ask a supportive friend with a great sense of humor to be in the room. Create an upbeat playlist, full of songs that unfold naturally. The more you can let your body go and trust the birth process and that your body and baby know exactly what to do, the more it will be able to relax. I remember years ago I worked with a woman who was set on her birth going a certain way. When things didn't go as planned, she held on so tightly and couldn't let go of control. She wasn't able to relax enough to let her cervix dilate.

No one ever knows how you're going to feel, act, or be until you're in that birth room. Birth has a way of bringing out all of your deepest fears, insecurities, vulnerabilities, repressed emotions, and wounds. It also brings out an enormous amount of love, power, strength, and courage.

---

lift your spirits. Use lavender to help you relax and destress, or maybe add some orange and ylang-ylang oil to your diffuser to uplift your spirit and lighten up the energy in the room.

I learned a valuable lesson from some of my teachers: When things get too heavy or serious, sometimes you just need to shake them up a bit by lightening the mood and having some fun so you can let go and shift the energy. I once had a client who wanted to feel supported and have her birth be light and fun. At one point we were playing dance music. We (myself, my client and her husband, the nurse, and the doctor) all started dancing and laughing. A few nurses down the hall peeked their heads in and, one by one, they all came in and joined the dance party. My client basically danced and laughed her baby down! By the time she was ready for pushing, she was so relaxed that she only had to push for a few minutes before her baby was in her arms and on her chest.

Another time, after 3 hours of pushing, one exhausted mother's husband lightened the mood by all of a sudden playing the song "Push It" by Salt-N-Pepa really loudly. We all started laughing and she got a second wind to keep going!

PAIN MANAGEMENT

Women's bodies and souls were created to do a lot of amazing things, and one of the most miraculous is to create, grow, and birth babies. Knowing this, I educate my clients by telling them the fewer medical interventions, the better for everyone. However, not everyone is down with going all natural. Again, everyone has different levels of coping and comfort.

If my client chooses to get an epidural, the only thing I ask is that they let me help them get to at least 4 to 6 centimeters dilated first. It used to be that 4 centimeters was considered active labor, but now many caregivers say that 6 is an optimal range for active labor. One of the reasons for holding off until around 4 if you can is that sometimes getting an epidural too early can slow down labor. After 6 centimeters, your body is in active labor and you will have less chance of needing other medical interventions. It also takes the longest time to get to 4 to 6 centimeters dilated; after that, labor tends to start moving faster. Keeping your body upright, either by walking, sitting on a birth ball, or kneeling against a sofa, helps gravity bring the baby down. Moving around freely, rocking, and changing positions will help to better align your baby for optimal fetal positioning for birth.

RIDING THE WAVES

Babies work so hard to be born. I always explain to my clients that they're helping their babies so much by just allowing their body to relax. You and your baby are totally in sync at birth—the two of you are the ultimate team. When a contraction happens, your baby is literally getting squeezed to life. The squeezing helps bring your baby down the birth canal and pump up her lungs, to get her ready to breathe on her own. The more you can relax into it and soften your body, the easier time your baby will have making her way down into your pelvis and out into the world.

Before you go into labor, it helps to start visualizing contractions as waves that come and go. You always want to be riding the contractions and going *with* them so they don't crash down on you and overtake you. Something to always remember is that these sensations you're feeling are your body doing *exactly* what it's meant to do. Often, when my clients acknowledge this powerful force inside them, thinking of it not as something happening outside of them but as their own body, it helps make the contractions more manageable. The more you can visualize your body opening instead of contracting, and flow with the waves instead of being overtaken by them, the easier time both you and your baby will have riding to the shoreline.

I help my clients ride the waves by walking them through each contraction, feeling it, breathing through it, and visualizing their baby corkscrewing down. As they relax during this process, not only are they helping their baby, but their cervix relaxes and opens. The more inward they go, the more intuitive and primal they become.

I also try different movements and positions with my clients and watch how their labor progresses with each. Sometimes I might just have a woman close her eyes, go within, and let her body quietly do what it needs and wants. One time, one of my clients starting crawling on the floor in between contractions and would go into Child's Pose and rock herself like a baby during the contraction. After it subsided, she would start crawling again. At one point she looked up and said, "I feel like I'm losing control." I told her not to worry, that I had her back and it was okay to let go. I assured her that she knew what to do! She just needed to trust herself, get out of her head, and let her body take over. Because she felt reassured that her behavior was perfectly natural, she was able to let go and continue laboring the way her body felt it should. Her baby happened to be spine to spine and she was experiencing strong back labor. Intuitively, she wanted to be on all fours crawling and rocking, which is the best position for back labor, since hanging forward takes the baby away from the spine and helps it turn. She didn't even know this at the time but, intuitively, when she let her body take over, it knew *exactly* what to do.

In order to get into the primal, intuitive groove of birth, you have to get out of your head and into your body. Some believe you should focus on something other than what's happening right here and now in your body. Go for a walk, do errands, eat, watch a movie—these are all great distractions for early labor. Staying busy is a great distraction while waiting for your labor to pick up.

When labor really starts going, I believe the only way "out" is to go "within." I do this by having my clients meditate and breathe into the contraction, sending healing breaths like they've been doing all along into their baby, and on the exhale opening their mouth and letting that sensation—whatever it might be— go through the breath as the belly softens and jaw relaxes, finally unclenching the cervix so the baby can corkscrew down and out.

In labor, there is a natural rhythm and flow. As you ride the waves of each contraction, you'll recognize that there's a natural space—a pause point—before the next one starts. I always think about surfing, when you paddle out to the break and wait until the wave comes before catching it to ride back to the shore. That space in between contractions is a very important time to rest. It's where you allow yourself to go within and regroup, recharge, and ground yourself before you exert a bunch of energy again to ride out that next wave of sensations. This will help pace your energy.

Ina May Gaskin, who has championed the use of midwives at births in the United States, says an open mouth equals an open cervix and an open throat equals an open vagina. She calls this the "sphincter rule."

Try this: Tighten your throat, clench your jaw, and purse your lips. Do you notice what happens to your lower belly and bottom? They naturally tighten up, which makes it very hard to labor and birth effectively. Ina May suggests kissing your partner passionately while in labor, because it loosens the mouth as well as the vaginal area. Kissing also releases oxytocin, which is great for relaxation.

Another thing I have my clients do during labor is open their mouths wide and yawn. This helps relax the lower belly and bottom. When you exhale during a yawn, you will also relax naturally.

SURRENDER TO THE NATURAL FLOW OF LABOR

I once was in labor with a client for 3 days. During her long labor, she went through a roller coaster of emotions. She came face to face with all of her fears, insecurities, and great discomforts. We worked through them one by one as they appeared, like hurdles she had to get past to advance. On her journey of letting go, these obstacles were stopping her from birthing not only her baby, but this new part of herself, as well. When she finally let them all go, her labor began to move and this force of strength, confidence, determination, and power came in as this new part of herself was emerging and being birthed.

You really need to be able to let it all go during labor. Penny Simkin, a doula and physical therapist who has specialized in childbirth education since 1968, often writes about how emotions can stall labor instead of allowing it to progress. If something comes up that you feel is stopping your labor from progressing, cry if you need to, talk about it, and let it out. Then, do breathwork to shift and clear this energy by breathing positive energy through your nose and exhaling the emotional energy out through your mouth. Take in what you need or want for support and let go of what you don't by talking and releasing the emotion. A few rounds of this breathing will shift your energy in a flash.

There is always a beginning and an end, a start and a stop. You can see this in the waves washing on the shore. Contractions are fluid movements that you can ride out like the waves that come and go on a beautiful shoreline. Say to yourself (or out loud): "With each contraction I ride I get closer to meeting my baby." The more relaxed you can be, the more relaxed your body will become, making it so much easier for your baby to make its way down and out into the world. Here are some things that promote relaxation.

- A peaceful and sacred birthing space
- A trusted, nurturing, and positive support system—a partner, doula, mother, sister, or loving friend
- Meditation and visualizations

BREATHE INTO YOUR BABY

Have your partner or doula place her hands or a warm water bottle on your belly. This helps give you a focus point to breathe into. It's also nurturing to have warm hands or something solid against you and supporting you. Breathe in the positive through your nose and exhale the negative out through your mouth. Breathe deeply right into your baby and let go through your mouth any fear or worry you might be feeling. Breathe into your baby the joy and excitement of meeting your baby and holding him in your arms soon, and exhale out through your mouth any impatience or frustration. Breathe in peace, calm, and relaxed energy to your baby, letting him know all is okay, and release any stress or tension through your mouth as your whole body relaxes. If you feel like it, on the exhale, give that sensation a sound—like an "ommmmm" or "ahhhhhh"—as you relax your jaw, neck, and shoulders, constantly letting that feeling go through your body by releasing the out breath through your mouth.

- Breathwork (like you've been taught throughout this book)
- Soft, soothing music
- Massage
- Gentle stroking of your head, back, or legs
- Water (take a shower or soak in the tub)
- Movement such as rocking and swaying in different positions
- Chanting
- Hypnotherapy
- Hugging or being held by your partner

Just as your child's birth will leave a lasting imprint on him, it will also leave a lasting imprint on you. With the right guidance and support, your birth can be one of the most beautiful, transformational, healing, and growing experiences you will ever have.

LABOR POSITIONS

One time, I was with a client during labor in the hospital. My client was 9 centimeters dilated and had had no medical intervention, except that she periodically wore a fetal monitor. I put my hand on her belly and I could feel her baby getting frustrated and pushing on her ribs like a springboard, trying to get down and out. I changed her position and had her do some deep, calming breathwork. As she breathed in through her nose, deep down into her baby, I had her exhale and totally relax her whole body. We then did the wave meditation. I could feel that the baby was now calm. A nurse came in and said, "Wow! Whatever you guys just did, it made this baby very happy. She was a bit stressed-out before!"

Below are some basic labor positions that I use a lot. There's no one perfect labor position for everyone, as everyone's body, baby

LABOR TIP: SQUATTING COUNTING

This is a great exercise to practice labor breathing and visualizations. You can breathe through anything for a 30-count breath. Imagine a line moving up as you count slowly to 15. Notice how it peaks, then count backward slowly from 15 to 1 as you visualize the line coming down the other side, like a mountain peak. This is how long a contraction usually lasts.

Lean with your back against a wall space with your feet hip-width apart, and place your hands at your sides. You can place a soft ball or a block between your thighs. Position your body as if you were sitting in a chair. When you start feeling a burning sensation in your legs, close your eyes, start to visualize the line, and count. When you get back to 1, stand up and take a break, then do a few more rounds. You can also have your partner count as you do focused breathing—inhale through your nose and exhale through your mouth as you relax out the burning sensation. Remember to count slowly and don't rush.

position, and labor are completely different. For example, I had a client whose labor was flowing beautifully as long as she was standing or kneeling. But whenever she sat down, her labor would stall, and if she lay down, it would stop. I always try a bunch of different poses and kind of sit back and watch how each pose affects my client and her labor. One person might love sitting on

BIRTH BALL BENEFITS

I'm also crazy about the birth ball for labor and highly suggest bringing one with you. Using a birth ball (a large exercise ball) has so many benefits! It opens and creates space in the pelvis, allowing your baby to drop down. Using a birth ball also helps speed up dilation, effacement, and the process of labor, and it relieves back, hip, and pelvic pain. After birth, it's awesome for soothing your baby by holding her as you sit

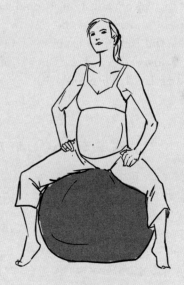

and bounce on it and to stretch out your chest, shoulders, and back, as well as to do core conditioning. I have clients who sit, rock, bounce, and move on the birth ball throughout their entire labor while I massage them and do energy work until it's time to push. When using the birth ball, it's important to recognize how your body feels, how your labor is going, and what you need. If labor is slowing down and you haven't slept, are exhausted, and need a little rest, step away from the ball for a bit, then get back into a position that gets things moving and grooving.

the birth ball, while someone else might hate it and prefer to lean on a couch instead. Try as many of these positions as you can and see what feels right for you and what works best for your labor and baby.

Standing is very productive in labor because it works with gravity, speeds up labor, and helps contractions become less painful. When you labor standing up, your baby becomes better aligned in the pelvis. Standing also oxygenates the baby.

Stair climbing can help your baby descend and speed up your labor. Climbing stairs works with gravity to help get your baby rotated into a good position for birth. It also helps open the pelvis and helps with mobility.

Walking and/or marching in labor is especially helpful in early labor as it helps gravity assist your body in getting your baby to move down into the pelvis.

Hip circles and swaying from side to side while standing help ease lower back and hip pain and feel good during a contraction or in between contractions. Imagine as you sway your hips from side to side and around that you're comforting and rocking your baby as he is getting squeezed by the contraction, rotating with ease further down into your pelvis.

Sometimes during a contraction you might need to hang on to a wall or chair, or you can throw your arms around your partner's neck and have him hug and hold you for extra support and TLC.

In a study from the *Journal of Perinatal Education*, researchers found mothers who stood up, walked around, or sat upright in the first stage of childbirth had a faster labor than those who lay down. In a related study from the *Journal of Midwifery and Women's Health*, women who walked around and were encouraged to change positions while in labor also had less of a need for pain medication during labor.

Lunging by placing a foot up on a chair helps the baby rotate as well as uses gravity to get the baby down. Stay in that position for a few contractions and then switch sides. This is also a nice stretch for tired or stiff legs.

Sitting is good for resting but still uses gravity to help drop the baby into the pelvis. I prefer the birth ball or a chair with pillows supporting your back. You can also sit facing the back of the chair—I like this position because your back can be massaged at the same time. You can also stack some pillows on a bed or couch and lean forward onto them. Again, this is great for getting a massage. Or have your partner sit behind you and lean into her, sitting up with your feet together and knees apart (Butterfly Pose); this helps open the pelvis. The toilet is also a great place to labor, although toilet contractions can be intense. But if you want to get that baby down and open things up, then I highly suggest sitting on the porcelain throne!

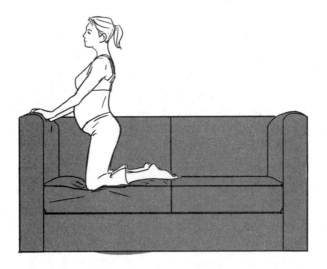

Kneeling is a great position I love, and so do many of my clients. Kneel on a couch facing the back, or kneel on a bed facing the headboard or wall. Place your hands up on the wall. You can even sway your hips from side to side during a contraction. Try kneeling, leaning on a birth ball, or a kneeling lunge— gravity helps the baby rotate during this position. Lunge on one side and then switch. Lunging while kneeling works as well as sitting and is similarly less tiring on the legs than walking or standing. Kneeling is also good when you need a break but still want to work with gravity to help move baby down and out.

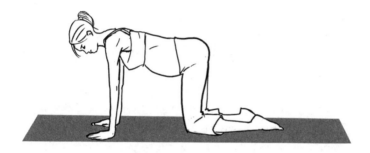

Getting on all fours is good for back labor. Being on your hands and knees helps shift and rotate baby away from your spine. And it helps relieve backaches. You can also try crawling on all fours or doing hip circles, hip swaying, or rocking back and forth while on all fours. And it's easy to go into Child's Pose from this position.

Squatting during pushing uses gravity and can help your baby descend into your pelvis. Squatting also increases the baby's rotation, is good for his circulation, and requires less bearing down when pushing. Like standing, squatting keeps baby well aligned with your pelvis. Try squats with a birth ball while holding hands with your partner, or have your partner sit behind you on the birth ball while you squat and lean on his legs.

Side lying is great for resting. It helps get more oxygen to the baby and lowers elevated blood pressure. Lying on your side

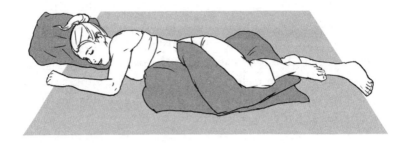

can slow a birth down that might be moving too fast, allowing you some time to rest in between contractions. Stack pillows between your knees to help open the pelvis. You can also place your top knee up on a table padded with pillows or in a hospital bed stirrup.

You can also do many of these positions (carefully) in the shower. Water is like a natural epidural and can really help with pain management. Allowing the water to fall on your lower back or belly is pure heaven for any laboring woman. Also, if your water hasn't broken, getting into a bathtub is ecstasy. I always turn to water when things really start moving. Water can change everything and make the whole process so much more manageable. I highly suggest at some point during the labor process getting into some water.

BIRTH AFFIRMATIONS

"Labor is the only blind date where you can be sure that you will meet the love of your life."

—Unknown

Birth isn't just a physical journey but a mental and emotional one, as well. The mind is a mighty powerful thing! In labor, your mind can be your greatest weapon and support, or it can sabotage your wishes and intentions, taking you down in the blink of an eye. Not everyone can have a doula's support throughout the birth process. When you have a doula by your side, she will be your greatest cheerleader—someone who lives, breathes, and speaks positive affirmations to you throughout the course of your labor.

I saw the idea of hanging up birth affirmations on a blog I read. I *love* this idea, and I now have all my clients make their own positive birth affirmations to hang up in the birth room as part of the sacred space I help create for them. I also encourage them to write the affirmations down to allow me or their support team to help with motivation by saying them out loud. During the birthing process, you may go through all kinds of emotional, mental, spiritual, and physical twists and turns and highs and lows. Birth affirmations will help support, ground, and focus your energy to help you stay strong and positive and have the birth you desire.

There are two ways you can make these affirmations. Use bright colors for both methods, since they tend to lift up the spirit, lighten the mood, and are more playful and cheerful to look at! I love this because it's like bringing the positive energy of all of the loved ones who support, care about, and nurture my clients into the birthing process.

As a baby shower ritual. On all the tables or on the walls of the room where you are having your baby shower, place large sheets of blank paper. Have colorful markers and crayons on the tables. Ask each of your guests to write out a positive birth affirmation for you and your baby-to-be.

Create your own. You can write out a list of your fears and turn those fears into a positive. For example, if your fear is, "I'm afraid I won't be able to do this," change it to, "My body is

Before birth, your body produces a hormone called relaxin, which softens your ligaments to help your baby pass through your pelvis during labor.

designed to do this" or "I'm strong and capable and trust my body to birth my baby with ease." I ask my clients when prepping them for birth, "What are some things I can say that will motivate you to give you more confidence and strength?" Or "How do you push yourself to get through a difficult physical exercise, challenging work project, or emotional experience?" If you're really creative, you can even draw out your birth intention with pictures, using words or feelings that inspire you. Pack some tape in your birth bag and hang your affirmations all over the walls and windows of your birth room.

Here's another way you can create these affirmations: Get a big jar or bowl (plain or decorated) and some paper or cute note cards. On the paper or cards, write as many positive intentions, quotes, prayers, mantras, poems, meditations, and affirmations as you can—anything that will support or empower you during the birth process. Or paste photos onto them. You can also ask your friends and family to add cards to the jar. Fill it up as much as you can. Bring the jar with you to the hospital. When you need a boost, pick a card out of the jar, read it, and enjoy.

Here are a few sample affirmations to get you started.

I am powerful.

There is no need to hurry.

I trust my labor process.

My body was made to do this.

I have all the time I need.

My body and my baby know exactly what to do.

I am a warrior.

I am a strong, capable woman.

My body contains all the knowledge necessary to give birth to my baby.

I trust my body to birth my baby.

Let go and relax.

I surrender with confidence.

I am safe.

I trust my intuition.

I trust my instincts.

There are 300,000 other women giving birth in the world with me today.

Every contraction brings me closer to meeting my baby.

The more I relax and let go, the easier time my baby will have making her way into the world.

I am a great mother.

I can do this.

I am committed.

No negative thoughts allowed in this room!

I breathe in relaxation, I breathe out tension.

I breathe love, peace, and joy into my baby and exhale fear, tension, or anxiety as my body relaxes.

I inhale oxygen and life force into my baby and, as I exhale, my whole body relaxes as my baby drops and my cervix dilates.

Breathe in "Let," exhale "go."

This present moment is all there really is.

I am fully here in the now.

There will be an end to this process where I will meet my baby.

The past is gone and the future hasn't happened yet.

What I do in this moment is building the way to my future.

You got this, girl!

LABOR AND DELIVERY CHECKLIST

These days, more and more women and couples are taking back the power of birth by voicing how they want their birth to be handled, as well as how they want themselves and their baby to be treated postbirth. Instead of allowing the medical professionals to follow their normal protocol, I always suggest doing your homework and researching *everything* first. Then, you can make educated choices when choosing your team and creating a birth plan. When you find what feels right for you, make sure you find a care provider who is on the same page and is supportive of your choices. Here's a basic list of caregivers and birthing options to consider. I purposely left out the pros and cons of each topic because I don't want to project my own views onto you and sway you in one direction or another.

- **Midwives** are trained professionals with expertise in promoting healthy pregnancies and supporting women throughout childbirth, recovery, and the postbirth period. Midwives are more likely to take a holistic approach with fewer interventions and to view your birth as a normal organic process (but they can give epidurals as well). Women who choose to be under the care of midwives tend to have a lower rate of C-sections. There are about 15,000 practicing midwives in the United States, and they are becoming more and more popular. Midwives practice in private homes, clinics, birthing centers, and hospitals. In many countries, midwives are the main health-care providers for women. They usually partner with a doctor in case there's any need of medical intervention, such as surgery.

- **Obstetricians** are the most common choice for medical care for pregnant women in the United States. An obstetrician is a doctor who specializes in pregnancy and birth. He or she has gone to medical school and is trained to handle every medical situation throughout pregnancy and birth. If you already see a trusted obstetrician and you like her bedside manner and philosophy on labor and birth, then sticking with that doctor may be the obvious choice for you.

- A **doula** is a woman who nurtures, supports, coaches, and guides women through pregnancy, childbirth, and the postpartum period. As I wrote in the introduction to this book, doulas advocate for their clients' needs and wishes. We don't deliver babies or perform any medical procedures. Doulas work with doctors and midwives as part of the birth support team no matter where and how their clients choose to give birth.

- **Hospitals** are, by far, the most popular location for giving birth. Hospitals are a more controlled and sterile environment in which to deliver a baby than a home, and many people feel safer having a baby in the hospital, knowing that medical intervention is right there if needed. If you choose an obstetrician as your caregiver, you'll most likely deliver your baby in a hospital with which he is affiliated. However, some doctors do deliver babies at birthing centers and, every so often, in homes. If you choose a hospital birth, go on a formal tour, speak with nurses and staff, read literature the hospital provides, and make sure the hospital policies meet your needs.

- A **birthing center** is a birthing facility with a more homelike feel that specializes in natural childbirth. If you're healthy, have a low-risk pregnancy, and want a more natural birth with no medical intervention and a more organic and familylike vibe (just not in your own home), a birthing center might be a good choice for you. Most birthing centers are linked with hospitals and doctors in case there is a need to transfer to a hospital.

- **Home birth** means laboring and birthing your child in the comfort of your own home. Home births are wonderful if you have a healthy and low-risk pregnancy, want to avoid any medical interventions, and want to enjoy the comforts of your home and familiar surroundings with your friends, family, and pets present.

- A **water birth** is just what it sounds like: giving birth to your baby in warm water. You can deliver in a bathtub, birthing tub, or other pool of water. You can have a water delivery at home, in a birthing center, or in a hospital. Water births are a popular choice since the baby has already been in amniotic fluid for 9 months. Birthing into a similar environment is a gentler way for the baby to come into the world as well as less stressful for the mother, as water helps tremendously with pain management.

- A **Caesarean birth (C-section)** is the surgical delivery of a baby, where the obstetrician makes an incision through the mother's abdominal wall and uterus to deliver the baby. C-sections are performed in an operating room and are considered major surgery. Generally, women are awake during the procedure but under regional anesthesia.

- **Natural childbirth** is a nonmedicated approach to laboring and birthing your child with very little to no medical intervention. Natural childbirth can take place at home, in a birthing center, or in a hospital.

- A **VBAC** is a vaginal birth after a Caesarean section. If you want to go for a VBAC, finding the right obstetrician or midwife who supports this decision is key.

- **Natural pain management** includes any nonmedical tactic to help with labor and delivery. Breathwork, massage, acupressure, acupuncture, movement, position changes, water, visualization, meditation, and birth under hypnosis are all things to learn about and add to your pain management repertoire.

- An **epidural** and a **walking epidural** are similar in that they are both used for medicated pain management during labor. The differences lie in both the procedure and the medications used. The walking epidural is a lower-dose epidural. It is a combination of spinal and epidural analgesia. The medications used are a local anesthetic and epinephrine, but in smaller amounts than in the regular epidural. You'll have more feeling in your lower body with a walking epidural, which is *very* helpful for moving around, changing positions, and pushing.

🖎 **Pitocin** is used in hospitals to help bring on or strengthen contractions during labor and delivery. Pitocin is the brand name for the drug oxytocin, a hormone found naturally in the pituitary gland. The drug is given intravenously and can be controlled as needed during labor and delivery. Pitocin can also be used to control bleeding after delivery and to help expel the placenta.

🖎 **Narcotics** are still given by some hospitals for pain management. Narcotics such as morphine, Demerol, and fentanyl, among others, help take the edge off pain and help women with contractions when they are trying to avoid getting an epidural. Taking these does have an effect on the baby.

🖎 **Circumcision** is something you will have to make a decision about if you're expecting a baby boy. Boys are born with a natural foreskin that covers and protects the head of the penis. In circumcision, the foreskin is surgically removed, exposing the end of the penis. For some, the choice to circumcise is based on cultural or religious beliefs.

🖎 **Cord blood banking** is another thing to consider. Cord blood is like liquid gold. It contains healing stem cells that can potentially help treat certain cancers and other conditions. There are several cord blood bank companies that you can research. For a fee, the company will send you a cord blood bank kit that you bring to the hospital or wherever you are delivering. Right after birth, your caregiver collects the blood in your baby's umbilical cord and placenta. You then call the cord blood bank and it will send a courier to pick up the package. It is then tested and stored in case you ever need it for medical use in the future. You can also donate your cord blood to a public bank that helps others in need.

🖎 **Cord tissue banking** is banking the tissue found in your baby's umbilical cord, which contains a special kind of stem cell different from the cord blood stem cells. These cells have the potential to rapidly regenerate and so can be useful in medical conditions that affect cartilage, muscle, and nerve cells.

🖎 **Delayed cord clamping and pulsating** refers to waiting for the cord to stop pulsating before cutting it. This is like giving your baby a megashot of iron and raises his hemoglobin levels as he transitions into life.

🖎 **Ingesting your placenta, or placenta encapsulation,** is the process of eating your placenta after birth. Ingesting the placenta has been shown to help with postpartum recovery by giving you energy, balancing your hormones, replenishing iron levels, increasing your milk supply, and warding off depression.

🖎 **Antibiotic eye ointment** such as erythromycin or tetracycline is given to babies within an hour after birth. The ointment is used to prevent newborn blindness from infection after birth, called ophthalmia neonatorum (ON). If the mother has a sexually transmitted disease (STD) such as gonorrhea or herpes, her baby is at higher risk for developing ON. You can request the gentler tetracycline drops or opt out altogether.

🖎 Since 1961, infants born in hospitals have received an **injection of vitamin K** into the leg muscle shortly after birth. This is not a vaccine, but a vitamin shot. It is given to prevent vitamin K deficiency bleeding (VKDB), a rare disorder that can occur because human infants do not have enough vitamin K, a blood coagulant, in their systems. Infants who develop VKDB can bleed in various parts of their bodies, including the brain. Less invasive oral doses of vitamin K are an alternative to the vitamin K shot. Some choose to opt out altogether.

🖎 The **hepatitis B** shot is another injection your newborn may receive after birth, either in the hospital or later, from your pediatrician. Hepatitis B is a viral infection that affects the liver. Infected women can pass on hepatitis B to their newborns.

Vaccines are a hotly debated topic among parents and doctors. It is a personal decision whether to vaccinate your child. Research and speak with several pediatricians before your baby is born to find out more about which vaccines are given when, what medication and other ingredients are in each vaccine, if they are really necessary, if they can be delayed and spread out over a longer period of time, and what they help to prevent.

IMPRINTING

Anyone who has worked with me knows how much I believe imprinting with a newborn is crucial for the bonding process to be successful. After all, the name of my pregnancy program is Rooted for Life! For me, pregnancy is all about creating a healthy foundation from which to grow, starting in the womb and continuing through the first year or so of your baby's life. It's this foundation that will lay the groundwork for the rest of her life! Up until now you were growing and building your baby. Just like a good builder uses the best materials to build homes, you've been eating better, thinking more positively, and feeling good about yourself as a mindful mom-to-be. In fact, the better care you take of yourself, the better your baby will feel and grow!

Imprinting at birth is so important! It's your child's first experience determining if this world is a safe and trustworthy place to be or not. All animals imprint with their babies. Birds use eye contact: When a bird is born, its mom looks straight into its eye so it imprints with and attaches to her. Sheep imprint by voice:

Touch is one of your baby's most advanced senses at birth. Even premature babies born as early as 25 weeks are aware of being touched.

Scientists in Norway videotaped babies who were delivered onto their mothers' tummies and found to their astonishment that, if left to their own devices, the babies used their limbs in a slow but coordinated way to crawl up and reach the breast, where they latched on and fed unaided.

"Baaahhhh" is all they have to say for that baby to know that this is his mother, even way out in the field with other sheep. Some animals lick and nuzzle their babies; others carry them around constantly until they're old enough to venture out on their own. Just as with animals, imprinting with our children right after their birth experience makes a big impact on them.

If you're having your baby at a hospital, ask the nurses to wait a few hours before doing any routine exams. Keep that baby on you, imprinting for at least a few hours. The first few hours post-birth is a magical time. This is the most awake your baby will be for the next few weeks, an important period to imprint and bond with you and your partner. Doing the following imprinting techniques will transition your baby into this world gently and help him feel that you have his back, that he's loved and safe in your arms and in this world.

Ways to Imprint with Your Child

I use the five senses to imprint, as these are all doorways to the soul. Just like we used the five senses in Chapter 7, when we worked on being present, take time to go inward with your baby now. Immediately after birth is the closest you'll ever see into your baby's soul! A midwife I work with suggests that all her clients turn the phones off. If you want a photograph, have someone else take it for you and wait a bit before texting, calling, and e-mailing everyone about the baby. This is such a magical and important time for you all as a family. Be present and unplug from the rest of the world, as you will never ever again have this moment with your child. I have my clients use all of the following imprinting techniques after birth.

❧ **Have skin-to-skin contact.** Babies thrive when they are returned to their natural habitat—their mother (or your partner if you are unable for whatever reason). Skin-to-skin contact is so important for newborns. If you can, hold your baby on your bare chest for as long as possible immediately after birth. Gently touch, stroke, kiss, and nuzzle your baby. This contact reassures the baby that she is in safe loving, hands. It also:

- Helps stabilize the baby's body temperature
- Stabilizes the baby's heart rate
- Normalizes the baby's breathing patterns
- Decreases levels of the baby's stress hormones
- Provides the comforting sound of your familiar heartbeat
- Exposes the baby to natural bacteria from you, which helps prevent sickness
- Increases the bonding process between mother and baby
- Makes the baby more likely to latch on to your breast right away, as well as feed longer and more easily. After your baby has been on you for a while, have your partner take off his shirt and do skin-to-skin contact next. This locks in the imprinting with him, too.

According to the *Journal of Psychological Science*, researchers made recordings of pregnant women reciting poetry and played them to babies in utero. When a baby listened to a recording of his mother's voice, his heart rate increased. The baby's heart rate would become slower when listening to a recording of another woman's voice.

- **Look your baby in the eyes.** They say the eyes are the windows to the soul and I must say I totally agree. I am always blown away when I look into a newborn's eyes as he first transitions to life in this world. I see something deeper than just his eyes—I am looking straight into his soul. It gives me chills just writing about it!

  We all have full access to this extraordinary window where you will see this little being in all his purity, light, and depth. When I prep someone for birth I always plant the seed of looking into her baby's eyes when he is first born. Looking lovingly into his eyes will not only allow you to really see him but will also help facilitate the imprinting, intimacy, and bonding process.

It's common to cut the umbilical cord between mom and newborn almost immediately after birth. Birth experts explain, however, that it's worth waiting for at least 90 seconds to 2 minutes, or until the umbilical cord stops pulsating, before cutting the cord. This is to allow the blood that is shared between the baby and your placenta to be completely absorbed by your newborn, giving her all of the nutrient-rich blood at birth.

I once asked Dr. Alan Greene, renowned pediatrician and author of *Raising Baby Green,* about waiting 90 seconds before clamping the umbilical cord and banking cord blood. He explained that cord blood banks prefer to bank cord blood when the umbilical cord pulsing slows rather than completely stops. After the cord stops pulsing, the blood can begin to clot quickly, which will interfere with collection. So, if you're planning on banking cord blood, consider waiting through a bit of pulsing before clamping the cord. He explains, "This treasure doesn't belong in the trash."

◈ **Talk lovingly.** Your and your partner's voices are already known to your baby. Your voices are what she's heard repeatedly throughout your pregnancy. Hearing your voice will comfort her after her big journey into the world! Speak to her from your heart, since babies are open vessels and can sense energy. Let your words hold the vibration of love and joy when your baby hears you for the first time from outside of your body.

◈ **Smell your baby's face and head.** There's a reason why your baby smells so good: A baby's head gives off love pheromones that help initiate the bonding process. In fact, researchers claim that a baby's smell lights up the same circuits in a mom's brain that good food does. It's a chemical communication that reaches both of you, right away, to allow you to bond with your newborn.

I'd also like to point out that if there was a complication at birth with baby or mom, please don't worry. You'll have plenty of time to make bonding memories with your little one. If you're unable to hold your baby after birth but your partner is, have your partner do skin-to-skin holding as soon as possible. When the time comes, you will have a lot of time to hold and bond with your baby skin-to-skin, talk to him, smell him, look him in the eyes, and imprint all your love onto him.

NEXT STEPS: HEALING

While you are getting used to the new addition to your family, you also need to pay close attention to your body. Some women bounce back very quickly after birth; others need some extra time to move and feel well again. I know I've said this a few times, but every woman's body responds differently to pregnancy and childbirth, and the same goes for healing and recovery postbirth. Don't compare yourself to anyone else. Tune in to what your own amazing body needs.

Lori's Postbirth Healing Pads

I make these pads in advance of my client's giving birth and have them ready in her home. They are easy to make (one batch makes a lot) and are completely natural. The cold from the freezer, combined with the healing ingredients, will help with the swelling and inflammation of your perineal area and will speed healing.

⅓ cup witch hazel, which helps with swelling and inflammation and helps fight bacteria on the skin

2 cups filtered water

1 dropperful liquid comfrey root, which is excellent for healing skin and is a natural topical pain reliever

10 drops liquid vitamin E oil, which brings moisture to the skin and has antioxidants to help with healing

10 organic minipads or panty liners (not too thick)

Dilute the witch hazel with the water in a jar with a lid. Add the liquid comfrey root and vitamin E oil. Close the jar and shake until blended well. Do not use the jar afterward for food, as comfrey should not be ingested.

Coat the entire surface of each panty liner with a thin layer of the mixture.

Wrap the liners individually in plastic wrap and place them in the freezer, laying them flat.

After your delivery, place a frozen pad in your underwear. Leave it in for 10 minutes, a few times a day.

If you have any liquid left over, put it in a clean squirt or spray bottle and spray your perineal area for additional relief after going to the bathroom or when using the shower.

Postbirth Sitz Bath

For a postbirth sitz bath, add flowers and herbs to help comfort your skin even more and speed up healing.

¼ cup lavender flowers

¼ cup calendula leaves

¼ cup comfrey leaves

3 cups Himalayan or Celtic sea salt

Mix together the lavender flowers, calendula leaves, comfrey leaves, and salt.

Add ½ cup of this mixture and ¼ cup witch hazel to warm bathwater. Stir the water and soak in the tub. Soak up to two times per day for 20 minutes total per day.

HEALING FROM A CAESAREAN SECTION

A C-section is a surgery that requires careful attention during healing. You will stay at the hospital longer than if you have a vaginal birth and your doctor will give you detailed instructions on how to heal. Your doctor will also want to see you often to make sure your body is healing well. My advice for women post C-section includes:

- Rest as often as you can! A good rule of thumb is to nap and sleep when baby naps and sleeps.

- Make sure you have people helping you and a good support team.

- Journal or talk to your partner, a friend, caregiver, or doula to process any disappointment you went through or are feeling postbirth. In my postbirth visit, I always recap the birth with my clients. It's very healing for the mom to talk about it.

- Take five arnica 30c pellets every 4 hours for the first few days to help with healing and soreness.

- Drink a mixture of comfrey and nettle leaf tea. Comfrey helps heal incisions and nettle leaf helps nourish you.

- Take 1 tablespoon of coconut oil before bed to help soften your stools. You won't be able to push or use your stomach muscles well, so you have to be careful what you eat.

PLACENTA ENCAPSULATION

In recent years I've seen more women ingest their placenta through a process called placenta encapsulation. The placenta is rich in nutrients that can help women recover from childbirth (both vaginal deliveries and C-sections). There are services that will take the placenta and process it into capsule form so you can take it like a vitamin. Here are some benefits of taking encapsulated placenta.

- Helps balance your hormones
- Replenishes depleted iron levels
- Assists the uterus in returning to its prepregnancy state
- Reduces postpartum bleeding
- Increases milk production
- Increases energy levels

THE 40-DAY RULE

Women in many cultures—Greek, Indian, African, and more—remain in their homes for the first 40 days after delivery. For the first 40 days after birth, your body is adjusting and replenishing itself. Your uterus is shrinking back to its normal size, you bleed on and off, and your body is healing and recovering from pregnancy and birth. It takes time to regain your energy and get "back to normal." If at all possible, I recommend following this rule to all my clients.

Staying inside for 40 days benefits both you and your baby. This is a sacred time to spend recovering from pregnancy and birth while getting to know, bond and connect with, and understand your baby. Now is also a good time to practice all of the tools you've been working on throughout your pregnancy. Here are some tips to help transition you and your baby, postpartum.

- Keep your support system going. Your partner, in-laws, friends, postpartum doula, or whoever has been helping you can now help out in other ways. Allow others to run errands, make meals, and do laundry so you can rest, recharge, and spend time bonding with your baby.

- The first 40 days can be both a restful and blissful time as well as a challenge, both physically and emotionally. Remember, your baby is new and also getting used to the world. You and your baby are trying to figure each other out and how things work. You only have this sacred time with your baby once in both of your lives, so take full advantage of it.

- Don't compare your experience to others'. I believe the same rules apply postbirth as during your pregnancy. Every woman has a different experience with her newborn and herself. Focusing on who has lost how much weight or whose baby is already sleeping well will add unnecessary stress during this time. Keep focused on yourself and your baby and you'll be a confident, empowered mom who knows she's doing the best for herself and her child.

NEXT STEPS: BREASTFEEDING

You're now starting to bond and connect with your baby. Somewhere between 36 and 72 hours after birth, your milk will begin to come in. This can be easy for some women but painful and uncomfortable for others. With practice and guidance, you can be on your way to successfully breastfeeding your newborn. Breastfeeding offers many benefits to both baby and mom.

For baby:

- Breast milk provides complete nutrition. It has a mix of vitamins, protein, and fat—everything your baby needs to grow.

- Breast milk is more easily digested than infant formula.

- Breast milk contains antibodies that help your baby fight off viruses and bacteria.

- Breastfeeding lowers your baby's risk of having asthma or allergies.

- Babies who are breastfed exclusively for the first 6 months, without any formula, have fewer ear infections, respiratory illnesses, and bouts of diarrhea.

- Physical closeness, skin-to-skin touching, and eye contact all help your baby feel secure.
- The American Academy of Pediatrics says breastfeeding also plays a role in the prevention of SIDS (sudden infant death syndrome).

For mom:

- Breastfeeding burns extra calories, so it can help you lose pregnancy weight faster.
- Breastfeeding releases the hormone oxytocin, which helps your uterus return to its prepregnancy size and may reduce uterine bleeding after birth.
- Breastfeeding also lowers your risk of breast and ovarian cancer, and it may lower your risk of osteoporosis.
- Breastfeeding saves you time and money, since you don't have to buy and measure formula, sterilize nipples, or warm bottles.

I always suggest asking for breastfeeding support at birth, whether that means seeing a separate lactation specialist or taking a breastfeeding class. Even if things seem to be going well in the feeding department, you want to make sure baby is latched on properly. For some women, breastfeeding is easy, and for others, breastfeeding can cause a lot of stress when baby isn't latching properly and getting enough milk. If for whatever reason you can't breastfeed, it's best to find a healthy alternative such as breast milk from a local milk bank or an organic formula to supplement breast milk. I've had clients who produce so much extra milk they donate it to others in need. If you aren't breastfeeding, you should still do skin-to-skin contact as often as possible when feeding.

Your newborn's stomach is only about the size of a cherry at birth, so he doesn't need very much to eat in the beginning (up to 1 ounce during each feeding for the first 3 days or so). Your colostrum, the "first milk" your body makes during pregnancy, will appear first. This will provide all the nutrients your baby needs before your milk comes in fully. Your baby may need to nurse frequently, which is helpful to both of you.

Here are some well-tested holistic remedies to help bring your milk down.

- Take sun chlorella, in either tablet or powder form. Sun chlorella enriches breast milk and also helps block environmental toxins from going to the baby through your breast milk.

- Have an alcohol-free beer. The hops in beer help produce more milk.

- Sleep. I know this is hard when you have a new baby, but try to sleep as often as you can when the baby sleeps.

- Nurse, nurse, and nurse some more. The more you nurse your baby, the more milk you'll make.

- Stay hydrated: Drink one 12-ounce glass of water every hour of the day. Always drink a glass while feeding your baby. Coconut water is also wonderful for hydrating yourself.

- Drink red raspberry tea. I like to make a pitcher of it, add some agave, fresh lemon, and mint, and have my clients drink it throughout the day. You can also drink mother's milk tea (but red raspberry tastes better).

- Take one to four capsules of fenugreek, three or four times per day. Fenugreek helps increase milk supply.

- Take four alfalfa capsules, three times a day. Alfalfa also helps enrich and increase breast milk supply.

Engorgement is the technical term for painful breasts due to milk that is there but isn't coming out very easily. Here are a few things you can do to help with engorgement.

- Nurse your baby as often as you can or, if you need to, pump as often as possible. This will kick-start your milk and allow it to flow better.

- Get in the shower and run hot water over your breasts. Let the milk just flow out, or you can do a gentle massage to help extract more milk or help it come in.

- Place a cool compress on your breasts after feeding.

HEALING NIPPLE BALM

If you're going to breastfeed, you'll be given a lot of help and advice about latching and nursing right away. When beginning to breastfeed, it's often normal for your nipples to get sore. Sometimes they even crack and bleed, becoming very uncomfortable. This is a great nipple balm that I make for my clients that helps protect nipples from cracking and drying out and helps heal them if they do. For my healing nipple balm, I use:

- 3 tablespoons calendula cream or ointment (repairs chapped or chafed skin)
- 3 tablespoons comfrey root ointment (heals cuts, burns, and abrasions)
- 5 drops vitamin E oil (promotes healing)
- 2 tablespoons lanolin (an anti-inflammatory, it moisturizes and speeds healing—just make sure you aren't allergic to lanolin before you add this!)
- 5 drops jojoba oil (moisturizes)
- 1 tablespoon cocoa butter (repairs, heals, and moisturizes)
- 1 teaspoon aloe vera gel (helps the skin repair itself)

I use a base of calendula cream or ointment and comfrey root ointment. Then, I mix in the rest of the ingredients. It's okay if you leave one of the moisturizers out or use more of one than another. Make sure everything is mixed well, and keep the balm in the refrigerator. (The cold feels good and soothing on the nipples, too.) Use the cream on your nipples liberally and as often as you need to. *Important: Be sure to wash your nipples before breastfeeding!*

After you wash off the cream, expose your nipples to sunlight and air for as long as you can (5 to 20 minutes). You don't have to be outside—just lie down or sit near a window. It's the perfect time for a catnap!

- Rub arnica oil over your breasts, but not on the nipples. Add a hot compress (hot towel, heating pad, or hot water bottle) to help soothe your breasts.

- Avoid tight-fitting bras or any clothing that is restricting.

This old wives' tale is actually true: You can place green cabbage leaves over your whole breast and in your bra between feedings. Cabbage is known to contain mustard oil, magnesium, oxalate, and sulphur heterosides, which have antibiotic and anti-irritant properties.

Wash a fresh head of green cabbage and place it in the refrigerator to chill. Slice off the tops of the "veins" with a sharp knife and cut several leaves to shape them to your breast. Drape one or two leaves over each breast, covering *all* of the engorged area. Leave the cabbage leaves on until they become wilted, about 20 to 30 minutes. Repeat three or four times within a 24-hour period, or until engorgement subsides. Use cabbage once in a while, since there's some thought that cabbage leaves can work *too* well and end up reducing your milk supply.

Lactation Smoothie

I have all of my clients make this smoothie during the first few weeks postbirth. The sun chlorella, almond butter, brewer's yeast, and oats help aid milk production.

1 frozen banana

⅓ cup rolled oats

1 tablespoon cacao powder

1 teaspoon sun chlorella powder

1 tablespoon brewer's yeast

1 tablespoon almond butter

½ cup almond milk

1 scoop protein powder

Ice to desired consistency

In a blender, combine the banana, oats, cacao, sun chlorella, brewer's yeast, almond butter, almond milk, protein powder, and ice. Blend until smooth.

Erica's Healing Stew

A good friend of mine and doula partner, Erica Chidi, is a maternity support specialist and founder of The Mama Circle in Los Angeles. This recipe is for her amazing stew that's perfect not only throughout pregnancy, but postbirth, as well. The yams and lentils are easily digested for a gentle meal, and the spices are mild yet flavorful and great for healing. It's also easy to prepare and takes no time at all to cook.

1 tablespoon organic coconut oil

2 tablespoons grated or finely chopped fresh turmeric

4 tablespoons grated or finely chopped fresh ginger

1 cup red lentils, rinsed and cleaned

5 garnet yams, peeled and coarsely chopped

6 cups organic chicken or vegetable stock

¼ cup organic coconut milk

1 bunch fresh cilantro, finely chopped

1 teaspoon salt

Black pepper to taste

In a large skillet or Dutch oven over medium heat, melt the coconut oil. Add the turmeric, ginger, and lentils. Cook, stirring frequently, for 3 to 5 minutes, until you smell the fragrant spices. Add the yams and mix until well coated and slightly caramelized.

Pour in the stock and bring to a gentle boil. Simmer over low heat until the lentils and yams are soft enough to mush with a spoon. Take the soup off the heat before you mix in the coconut milk and cilantro.

Season with the salt and black pepper to taste.

BIRTH PLANS

"The question is not whether women have a choice, but are they willing to make a choice."

—**Kim Wildner**

You've just read about going with the flow and letting go of control. When you think about giving birth, I always recommend having a plan or a more relaxed way to map out your labor and birth intentions. There are a lot of factors to consider during labor and delivery.

I worked with a woman once who was a little *too* "go with the flow" about her birth options and said the doctors and nurses could do whatever they wanted with her and her baby during labor. I sat her down and had her fill out a birth plan. I asked her, would you really be okay if they did this to you or that to your baby? Needless to say, the answer was no! This is one way to take back some power in birth, especially in a hospital setting. Women have so many choices about giving birth and how to bring babies into this world. If we don't know and state our needs and options, those choices can be taken away very quickly.

Birth plans are great tools to help prepare for and educate yourself about birth. They get everyone on the same page (*your* page). Birth plans help express the way that you want to be treated and the way you want your birth and baby to be handled. Without knowing what your wishes are, the hospital will use protocol.

This is a basic birth plan. I've tried to cover all aspects of labor and delivery that you may face, whether in a hospital, birthing center, or at home. Read through it and think about every part of the plan. You may change your mind about certain things as your pregnancy—or even labor—progresses. The most important thing is that you research all your options, educate yourself in all your choices, and are comfortable with what you have chosen.

Here are some questions I ask my clients prebirth to gain a deeper understanding of how they operate and how I can best support them. You might want to answer and share them with your birth partner, doula, or team.

- What helps you feel better if you are nauseous, sick, or achy?
- What helps you feel safe and calm when you are experiencing or doing something new?
- When experiencing a painful situation, do you tend to go more inward or seek soothing and support from others?
- How do you tend to handle pain?
- When you feel scared, what most helps you to feel safe?
- When you are stressed-out, what techniques have you found to help you relax and be calm? For example, do you turn to massage, meditation, or some other relaxation tool?
- What are some things you tell yourself to push yourself through heavy physical exertion or when you're trying to reach a goal? Make these birth affirmations.
- What kind of touch relaxes you the most? On your hands, feet, or head?
- Are there certain aromatherapy oils you prefer and any that you dislike?
- What kind of music do you like?

- Are there any negative, doubting voices in your head (either your own or your projection of other people's) that might get in the way of obtaining your birth goal? If so, what are they?

I also ask the following questions about possible past traumas. The reason I ask these questions is because in birth a flashback, feeling, or deep-seated fear from a past trauma can possibly resurface.

- What was your mother's birth with you like?
- Have you experienced any traumatic event in the past (death of a close friend or relative, accident, sickness, etc.)?
- Have you ever had a traumatic experience in a hospital?
- If you have had other children, what was your birth like with them?

MY BIRTH PLAN

FULL NAME

PARTNER'S NAME

BABY: BOY   GIRL   UNKNOWN

TODAY'S DATE

DUE OR INDUCTION DATE

ADDRESS

E-MAIL

DOCTOR OR MIDWIFE

HOSPITAL, BIRTHING CENTER, OR HOME

I WOULD LIKE THE FOLLOWING PEOPLE TO BE PRESENT FOR THE LABOR AND/OR BIRTH OF MY BABY (write out names):

PARTNER

FAMILY

FRIENDS

DOULA

CHILDREN

OTHER

PLEASE DO NOT ALLOW

Hospital Birth

PLEASE NOTE (check all boxes that apply):

☐ I am pregnant with twins.

☐ I am Rh-negative.

☐ I have group B strep.

☐ I have gestational diabetes.

☐ I eat a special diet of _____.

☐ Because of religious reasons, I _____.

☐ I am allergic to _____.

☐ I am currently taking these medications: _____.

☐ Other (example: I suffer from anxiety): _____

_____

DURING MY LABOR, I WOULD LIKE/PREFER (check all boxes that apply):

☐ To have the option of going home if I am less than 4 centimeters dilated

☐ To stay at the hospital no matter how dilated I am

☐ That no residents or students assist with or attend my birth

☐ To listen to music

☐ To have dimmed or natural lighting

☐ To wear my own clothes

☐ To wear hospital clothing

☐ To have my partner present the whole time

☐ To have the room as quiet and peaceful as possible

☐ To have as few interruptions as possible

☐ To wear my contacts or glasses

☐ To take pictures and/or make a video during labor and birth

☐ To hydrate with clear fluids instead of having an IV

☐ To have a heparin or saline lock

☐ To walk around and move freely

☐ To eat

☐ To have intermittent fetal monitoring

☐ To have continual fetal monitoring

☐ To keep my door closed

☐ To have as few vaginal exams as possible

FIRST STAGE OF LABOR

DURING THIS STAGE, I WOULD PREFER TO:

- ☐ Walk and move around, getting into different positions
- ☐ Lie down
- ☐ Sit on a birth ball
- ☐ Take a shower
- ☐ Take a bath

PAIN RELIEF:

- ☐ We are having natural childbirth and will not need pain relief.
- ☐ Please only provide pain relief if I ask for it.
- ☐ If you see I am in pain, please suggest options to me.

I WOULD LIKE TO TRY THESE NATURAL METHODS FOR PAIN RELIEF:

- ☐ Breathwork
- ☐ Water (bath or shower)
- ☐ Sound therapy
- ☐ Movement
- ☐ Massage
- ☐ Acupuncture
- ☐ Acupressure
- ☐ Hypnotherapy
- ☐ Visualization
- ☐ Meditation
- ☐ Distraction techniques
- ☐ Heat and cold therapy
- ☐ Reflexology
- ☐ Aromatherapy

IF I DO CHOOSE MEDICAL PAIN RELIEF, MY PREFERENCE IS:

- ☐ Walking epidural
- ☐ Classic epidural
- ☐ Sedative
- ☐ Narcotics

I WOULD LIKE TO USE OR BRING THE FOLLOWING LABOR PROPS:

- ☐ Body pillow
- ☐ Birth ball
- ☐ Squat bar (most hospitals have this)
- ☐ Tub
- ☐ Birthing stool
- ☐ Other _____

SECOND STAGE OF LABOR

I WOULD LIKE TO USE THESE POSITIONS FOR PUSHING AND BIRTHING
MY BABY:

☐ Squatting

☐ Semireclining

☐ Lying on my side

☐ Getting on all fours

☐ Kneeling lunge

☐ Birthing stool

☐ Standing

☐ Whatever feels right for me at the time

EPISIOTOMY:

☐ I prefer not to have one and will risk tearing.

☐ Please only perform an episiotomy using local anesthesia or pressure.

TO HELP PREVENT TEARING, I WOULD LIKE THE FOLLOWING:

☐ To have a hot compress applied

☐ To have perineal massage

☐ To have oil applied

☐ To breathe through a slower crowning

WHEN IT'S TIME TO PUSH:

☐ I would like to do so instinctually, when I have the urge.

☐ I want to be coached on when to push.

☐ I want a combo of instinctual and coached pushing.

☐ I want to have unlimited time, as long as my baby and I are okay.

☐ If I get an epidural, I would like it to wear off while pushing.

☐ I want to use a mirror to see the birth of my baby.

☐ I want to touch my baby's head as it crowns.

☐ I want to avoid vacuum extraction.

☐ I prefer that the doctor catch the baby and place him/her on my chest.

☐ I prefer that my partner catch the baby and place him/her on my chest.

☐ I would like to catch my baby and pull him/her onto my chest.

☐ I prefer that the room be silent and that our voices be the first sound the baby hears.

☐ I prefer the use of dim or natural lighting for the birth.

AFTER BIRTH:

☐ I want to hold my baby and have skin-to-skin contact right away.

☐ I want to cut the cord and bank the cord blood.

☐ I am banking both cord blood and cord tissue.

☐ I want to allow the cord to pulse for 30-60 seconds before cutting and then bank the rest.

☐ I wish for the cord to remain attached until it stops pulsating.

☐ I want to donate cord blood.

☐ I want my partner to cut the cord.

☐ I want to deliver the placenta spontaneously, without Pitocin.

☐ I want to save my placenta and take it home with me.

☐ I want to breastfeed right away when the baby starts rooting.

IF HAVING A C-SECTION:

☐ My partner/doula is to be present at all times during the operation.

☐ Please lower the screen so I can see my baby being delivered.

☐ I would like to remain as conscious as possible during delivery.

☐ Please discuss anesthesia options with me.

☐ I would like the surgery explained as it is happening.

☐ I would like the baby to be shown to me, to have eye contact with me, and to be placed on my chest for skin-to-skin contact in the operating room immediately after delivery.

☐ I would like the birth to be photographed.

☐ I would like to play my own music.

☐ I ask for the room to be quiet and that those present please avoid small talk.

☐ I would like for my partner to hold the baby and have skin-to-skin contact as soon as possible.

IN RECOVERY:

☐ I want to breastfeed and have skin-to-skin contact right away.

☐ If my baby needs additional medical attention, my partner needs to be with my baby at all times.

EXAMS AND PROCEDURES (FOR BABY):

☐ Hold off until after we've had some time for bonding.

☐ Perform exams and procedures in either my or my partner's presence.

☐ My pediatrician will give _____ to my baby.

    ☐ Heel stick for screening tests beyond the PKU test

    ☐ Hepatitis B vaccine

    ☐ Hearing test

    ☐ Vitamin K: ☐ shot or ☐ oral

    ☐ Antibiotic eye ointment

    ☐ A bath

☐ Please use my products that I brought to bathe my baby.

☐ Please bathe the baby in my or my partner's presence.

☐ Please don't bathe my baby, and leave vernix on.

FEEDING:

☐ I plan on breastfeeding exclusively.

☐ Please offer assistance for lactation support.

☐ I plan to combine breastfeeding and formula.

☐ I plan to feed formula only.

☐ Please only use this formula that I brought with me: _____

☐ Please don't give my baby formula.

☐ Please don't give my baby sugar water.

☐ Please don't give my baby a pacifier.

IF I HAVE A BOY, CIRCUMCISION:

☐ Should not be performed

☐ Should be performed by _____

☐ Will be performed later

☐ Should only be done in the presence of me or my partner

☐ Should be performed with anesthesia

I WOULD LIKE MY BABY TO STAY IN THE ROOM:

☐ 24 hours a day

☐ Unless I ask for the baby to go to the nursery

HOSPITAL STAY:

☐ I would like to leave as soon as possible.

☐ I would like to stay as long as possible.

SPECIAL REQUESTS, QUESTIONS, AND NOTES FOR YOU, YOUR PARTNER, OR YOUR DOCTOR:

_____

_____

_____

_____

_____

_____

_____

_____

_____

_____

_____

_____

_____

_____

Home Birth

I usually don't make birth plans for home births because midwives are on the same page for a natural birth and there is no hospital policy. However, filling out a birth plan is a good idea in case you need to be transferred to a hospital.

FIRST STAGE OF LABOR

☐ I would like to remain as active as possible, finding the best positions for myself and changing these as I wish.

☐ I would like to try to rest between contractions when possible.

☐ I would like monitoring of the baby to be kept to a minimum unless there is cause for concern.

☐ I would like intervention, such as breaking of my water, to be kept to a minimum.

I WOULD LIKE TO TRY THESE NATURAL METHODS FOR PAIN RELIEF:

☐ Breathwork

☐ Water (bath or shower)

☐ Sound therapy

☐ Movement

☐ Massage

☐ Acupuncture

☐ Acupressure

☐ Hypnotherapy

☐ Visualization

☐ Meditation

☐ Distraction techniques

☐ Heat and cold therapy

☐ Reflexology

☐ Aromatherapy

TRANSITION:

☐ I want to be very centered on myself at this stage and to have no intrusions.

☐ Please give me gentle support and firm guidance.

☐ Please keep me informed on my progress.

SECOND STAGE OF LABOR

I WOULD LIKE TO USE THESE POSITIONS FOR PUSHING AND
BIRTHING MY BABY:

☐ Squatting

☐ Semireclining

☐ Lying on my side

☐ Getting on all fours

☐ Kneeling lunge

☐ Birthing stool

☐ Standing

☐ Whatever feels right for me at the
time

WHEN IT'S TIME TO PUSH:

☐ I would like to do so instinctually, when I have the urge.

☐ I want to be coached on when to push.

☐ I want to have unlimited time, as long as my baby and I are okay.

☐ I want to use a mirror to see the birth of my baby.

☐ I want to touch my baby's head as it crowns.

☐ I prefer that the midwife catch the baby and place him/her on my chest.

☐ I prefer that my partner catch the baby and place him/her on my chest.

☐ I would like to catch my baby and pull him/her onto my chest.

☐ I prefer that the room be silent and that our voices be the first sound the
baby hears.

☐ I prefer the use of dim or natural lighting for the birth.

☐ We plan to take photographs or videotape the birth.

☐ We want to discover the sex of our baby ourselves.

☐ If I do tear and stitching is necessary, I do want a local anesthetic to be
administered beforehand.

BIRTH ROOM(S):

☐ I intend to use the _____ room(s) for birth. The birthing pool will be in the _____ room.

☐ There will be special lighting/music/scents.

☐ There will be a bright, poseable lamp available for the midwives' use.

☐ My other child(ren) will have someone taking care of them and may come in and out of the room at appropriate times.

☐ My child(ren) may want to watch the delivery.

☐ Food and drink for midwives and helpers will be available in the _____ room.

EMERGENCIES:

In case of an emergency, it's always good to have the Hospital Birth plan filled out as well, to establish the way you want to be treated and your birth to be handled once you get there.

☐ My partner and I will discuss situations as they arise. Please share any concerns with us as soon as they arise. It will help us to know the answers to these questions:

1. What's wrong?

2. What do you suggest and why?

3. What are the possible outcomes with and without this intervention?

4. How much time do we have to make a decision?

5. Are any other courses of action open to us?

☐ If we go to the hospital, I would like my partner and my support team to be with me.

☐ In the event that a C-section is necessary, I would like to have a spinal/ general anesthetic.

AFTER BIRTH:

☐ I want to hold my baby and have skin-to-skin contact right away.

☐ I want to cut the cord and bank the cord blood.

☐ I am banking both cord blood and cord tissue.

☐ I want to allow the cord to pulse for 30–60 seconds before cutting the cord and then bank the rest.

☐ I wish for the cord to remain attached until it stops pulsating.

☐ I want to donate cord blood.

☐ I want my partner to cut the cord.

☐ I want to deliver the placenta spontaneously.

☐ I want to keep my placenta.

☐ I want to breastfeed right away when the baby starts rooting.

SPECIAL REQUESTS, QUESTIONS, AND NOTES FOR YOU, YOUR PARTNER, OR YOUR MIDWIFE:

_____

_____

_____

_____

_____

_____

_____

_____

_____

_____

_____

ACKNOWLEDGMENTS

I'd like to thank all the amazing moms and moms-to-be I have worked with over the years! Each one of you has taught me something new. Even though you hired me to guide and support you, you have all been invaluable teachers to me. I could not have written this book or been able to share this information without all of you!

I want to thank my parents for always supporting me to be myself and for believing in me. For all of their constant love and encouragement, my friends (too many to name, but you all know who you are) are huge blessings in my life. I want to thank all of my teachers, including Michele Meiche, Seane Corn, and Peter Evans, for helping me heal and become the person I am today. A little extra shout-out to Michele Meiche, because I would not be writing and aligned to my soul's path if it wasn't for your constant nudging and guidance.

Thank you to my cowriter, Stefani, for putting up with me, my disorganized e-mails, crazy messages, for keeping me on track and putting in so many long hours. Your help writing this book was beyond priceless! To my awesome literary agent, Brandi Bowles, for seeing something special and taking a chance on me. To my fabulous editor, Ursula Cary Ziemba, for always being so excited, supportive, and positive. You made this whole journey of writing a book easy and drama-free! Thanks also to the rest of the amazing team at Rodale Books. I'm so blessed to have you all in my life.

With deep love and gratitude,
xo Lori

INDEX

Boldface page references indicate illustrations. Underscored references indicate boxed text.

Drinks *(cont.)*
  for constipation relief, 100
  DIY Pregnancy Tea, <u>119</u>
  Elissa Goodman's Iron Juice, <u>121</u>
  Lactation Smoothie, <u>277</u>
  Lori B's Fabulously Yummy
    LaborAde, <u>235–36</u>
  Mood-Boosting Smoothie, <u>167</u>
  for muscle cramp alleviation, 141,
    142
  My Favorite Go-To Constipation
    Cocktail, <u>102</u>
  teas, 86, 119–21
  water, <u>9</u>, 38, <u>39</u>, 97, 201
Due date, 2, 211–12
Duration of pregnancy, 2

E

Eating. *See* Diet and food
Edema or swelling, 216–17, <u>220</u>
EFAs, 10–11, <u>94</u>
Electrolytes, replenishing, 100
Embracing your authentic self
  both strengths and weaknesses,
    63–64, 74–75
  Burning Man inspiring, 75–77
  creating a picture, 77, 79
  "hats" of self-expression, 71–72
  journaling, <u>78</u>
  masks concealing yourself, 72–73
  parenting and, 64–65, 69–71
Emotional alarms, 42–44
Emotions. *See also* Fear and worries;
    Stress
  being present with, 177–78
  distracting ourselves from, 177
  mood-boosting foods, <u>101</u>
  Mood-Boosting Smoothie, <u>167</u>
  mood swings, 34–35
  morning and evening transitions,
    45
  trigger, 42, <u>46</u>
Energy
  bringing to the present, 183–84
  conserving during labor, 214
  diet for, 86
Energy leaks, 192
Engorgement relief, 275, 277

Entrées
  My Healthier Mac and Cheese,
    <u>51</u>
  My Mama's Lasagna, <u>236–37</u>
Environment. *See* Green living
Epidural, 246, 262–63
Episiotomy, 194–95, 213–14
Essential fatty acids (EFAs), 10–11,
    <u>94</u>
Essential oils
  for birthing, 199
  for at-home spa, 59–60
  Love Soak Bath Meditation, <u>221</u>,
    <u>223</u>
  in recharging bath, 60
  for starting labor, 227
Estrogen. *See* Hormones
Exercise. *See also* Yoga
  back pain and, 128
  brain development and, <u>171</u>
  for carpal tunnel syndrome, 167
  gentle, 193
  guidelines during pregnancy, 18
  health benefits of, 17
  Kegel exercises, 81–82, 201
  labor stimulated by, 227
  listening to your body, 17, 18
  for muscle cramps, 142
  starting slowly, 17
  for varicose veins, 179
Exercises. *See also* Breathing;
    Journaling
  being present, 173
  body scan, 57–59
  bringing your energy to the
    present, 183–84
  calling in your baby, 3–4
  inner child conversation, <u>160–62</u>
  letters to your baby, 4–5, 134
  Love Soak Bath Meditation, <u>221</u>,
    <u>223</u>
  picturing your authentic self, 77,
    79
  "plucking out the weeds"
    meditation, 206–7
  recharging bath meditation, 60
  shifting energy, 73–74
  squatting counting, <u>251</u>
  tantric relationship bonding
    meditation, <u>159</u>, 163

Intuition *(cont.)*
    "I feel you" letter, 134
    as inner guru, 124
    in naming your baby, 134–35
    tapping into, 123, 125
    thinking vs., 126, 130–31
    three voices exercise, 130–31
    trusting yours, 123–24, 125
Inventory of your life, taking, 191
Iron
    checking your levels at home, 87
    deficiency (anemia), 11, 83–84
    with delayed cord clamping and
        pulsating, 264
    Elissa Goodman's Iron Juice, 121
    foods high in, 11, 84–86

J

Journaling
    adjustments based on, 15–16
    finding perfection in
        imperfection, 243
    food log, 14–16
    getting fears out, 244–45
    identifying your stress, 98–99
    parenting yourself Q&A, 46–48
    patching up issues within, 151
    practicing gratitude, 222
    questions to answer, 15
    three voices exercise, 130–31
    on your authentic self, 78
Joy list, 47

K

Kegel exercises, 81–82, 201, 217
Kicking. *See* Movement by baby
Kitchen, preparing for baby, 191
Kneeling in labor, 254–55, **254**

L

Labor. *See also* Birth
    birth ball for, 252, **252**
    body awareness before, 223–25
    checklist, 260–65
    fear about pain, 213

    fetal positioning for, 226
    getting it started, 226–27
    pain management, 246
    pooping while pushing, 213
    positions, 210, 247, 251–56, 253,
        254, 255, 256
    riding the waves, 246–48
    squatting counting exercise, 251
    start of, 212–13
    surrendering to the flow of,
        249–50
    time required for, 218–19
    trusting the process, 241
Legs on the Wall Pose, 23, **23**
Lemon Ice Cubes, 53
Length of pregnancy, 2
Lentils, 101
Letters to your baby, 4–5, 134
Lizard Pose, 118, **118**
Low Lunge, 117–18, **117**
Lunging in labor, 254

M

Marching in labor, 253
Masks concealing yourself, 72–73
Massage
    for conditions
        back pain, 128
        carpal tunnel syndrome, 166,
            167
        constipation, 101
        edema, 217
        muscle cramps, 141–42
        varicose veins, 179–80
    foot, 184
    perineal, 194–95
Maternity clothes, 28
Meditations. *See* Exercises
Midwives, 260
Minerals
    calcium, 10
    iron, 11, 83–86, 87, 121, 264
Mold-killing spray, 29
Mood-boosting foods, 101
Mood swings, 34–35
Morning sickness. *See* Nausea or
    morning sickness

R

S

Sacred space, creating, 196–200
Scrub, lemon-sugar, <u>61</u>
Seated Cross-Legged Forward Bend
 with Chair, <u>55</u>, **55**, <u>114</u>, **114**
Seated Forward Bend with Chair,
 <u>140</u>, **140**
Senses
 connecting to the now, 174–76
 hearing, baby's, 129, 132–33
 sight, baby's, <u>171</u>
 sound of your voice, 132–33, 172,
  <u>174</u>, <u>267</u>, 269
 taste, baby's, 154
 touch, baby's, 154, 176, <u>177</u>, <u>265</u>
 walking meditation on, 180–81
Sex, 82–83, 226
Shoes, leaving outside, 28
Shower, baby, affirmations at, 257
Side dish
 Roasted Root Veggies, <u>187</u>
Side lying in labor, 255–56, **256**
Side Stretch, <u>139</u>, **139**
Sight, 68–69, <u>171</u>, 175
Simple Seated Breathwork, <u>224</u>, **224**
Sitting in labor, <u>253</u>, 254
Sitz bath, 201, <u>270–71</u>
Skin, baby's, 128, <u>129</u>
Skin, yours
 acne, 108–10, <u>110</u>
 itchy, 171
 Simple Lemon-Sugar Scrub, <u>61</u>
 Soothing Lavender Face Mask,
  <u>61</u>
Skin care products, 25
Skin pigmentation, changes in, 90
Skin-to-skin contact, 267
Sleep
 by baby, <u>196</u>
 back pain and, 127
 fatigue from too little, 36–37
 muscle cramps and, 142, 143
 stretches before, 144–45
 sweating during, 40
 transitions to and from, 45,
  48–50
Smells, <u>146</u>, 175–76, <u>176</u>, 269

Song of the baby, <u>135</u>
Soup
 Erica's Healing Stew, <u>278</u>
 Stefani's Hand-Me-Down
  Chicken Soup, <u>165</u>
Spa, at-home, 59–60
Sphincter rule, <u>248</u>
Spinach, 88
Sprays, <u>29</u>, <u>215</u>
Squats, <u>106–8</u>, **106**, **107**, **108**, 226
Squatting counting exercise, <u>251</u>
Squatting in labor, 255
Stair climbing in labor, 253
Standing Calf Stretch, <u>144</u>, **144**
Standing in labor, 253, <u>253</u>
Starting labor, 226–27
St. John's wort oil, <u>179</u>
Stress. *See also* Fear and worries
 effect on your baby, 93–95, <u>93</u>,
  96
 fish for lowering, <u>94</u>
 identifying your stress, <u>98–99</u>
 symptoms of, 95–96
 tips for stress relief, 96–97
 yoga for stress relief, 110–15
Stretches. *See* Yoga
Stretch marks, preventing, 79–80,
 <u>80–81</u>
Supplements
 alfalfa, <u>36</u>, 97, 100
 antioxidants, 11
 constipation-relieving, 97, 100
 fatigue-fighting, 37, 53
 folic acid, 12, <u>12</u>
 hemorrhoids-relieving, 201
 powdered greens, 10
 primrose oil, <u>235</u>
 probiotics, 9–10
 for varicose veins, 179
 vitamin D, 8–9
 vitamin E, 9
Supported Bridge Pose with Block,
 <u>105</u>, **105**
Supported Fish Pose, <u>203</u>, **203**
Supported Side Stretch, <u>185</u>, **185**
Surrendering to the flow of labor,
 249–50
Swaying in labor, 253